50 THINGS THAT CAUSE OBESITY

Dr Ashish Indani

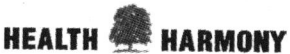

An imprint of
B. Jain Publishers (P) Ltd.
USA — Europe — India

> **Disclaimer**
>
> Any information given in this book is not intended to be taken as a replacement for medical advice. Any person with a condition requiring medical attention should consult a qualified practitioner or therapist.

50 THINGS THAT CAUSE OBESITY

First Edition: 2012
1st Impression: 2012

All rights reserved. No part of this book may be reproduced, stored in a retrieval system or transmitted, in any form or by any means, mechanical, photocopying, recording or otherwise, without any prior written permission of the publisher.

© with publisher

Published by Kuldeep Jain for

HEALTH HARMONY

An imprint of
B. JAIN PUBLISHERS (P) LTD.
1921/10, Chuna Mandi, Paharganj, New Delhi 110 055 (INDIA)
Tel.: +91-11-4567 1000 • *Fax:* +91-11-4567 1010
Email: info@bjain.com • *Website:* **www.bjain.com**

Printed in India by
J.J. Offset Printers

ISBN: 978-81-319-0848-8

Preface

The uneven distribution of fats in the body of an individual, called obesity, is a hefty problem, which is turning almost to an endemic all over the world. It is a major issue in respect to health care domain. Not only in the Middle East and in the American countries, but also in Asia and the European countries – the prevalence of the overweight tendency and obesity is very high. With the growing modernisation of several societies globally, the diet and exercise habits are modified in particular, adversely, which conveniently ignores the balance between exercise, diet intake and climatic energy requirements.

A surprising point here is that most of us are quiet indifferent to the obese constitutions.

In spite of the mushrooming of weight reducing services and products, over last one decade, obesity is growing with a steep statistical curve. A classical concept of overeating effect is also exploited beyond actuals and in most cases, there is more of panic than practical and scientific discussions. Other causes of obesity such as subclinical hormonal imbalance and dietary deficiencies are often ignored. Efforts of the people in reducing weight and keeping themselves fit is also exponential in reference to the period. Lack of motivation, attachment to taste and cultural obsessions about eating habit are the largest contributors to this indifference.

When Dr Geeta discussed the topic of this short book on obesity with me, I was pleased to contribute my research outcomes and several understandings on this front. I decided to go with all what I had done for my project once again. Revised knowledge from several books, internet information sources, practical experience in clinic and research experiences in my own and my intern's projects, was my major source for information. This whole information is presented in scientific but simple form for you to get practical tips about your weight management and to keep fit.

Acknowledgements

First of all, I thank my spiritual masters and my source of inspiration, His Holiness Rangunathji (Paresh Kumarji) Goswami, His Holiness Radhanath Swami, His Holiness Loknath Swami and His Grace Sikshashtaka Prabhu. My sincere thanks to my family – to my father, Omprakash Indani; to my mother, Mrs Uma; to my wife, Dr. Aashlesha; sister, Ms Sneha and grandmother, Kamala Indani. I thank my colleague for – Projects on obesity, especially the ASSOIL-Intake trial; my wife and co-investigator Dr Aashlesha; my friends and sub-investigators Mrs Roshika Banerjee, my friends and the surveying team Mr Rajbir Sandhu, Mr Arbaz Shaikh, Mr Alnavaz, Ms Aayushi Modi, Mr Bhavesh Hapani, Mr Kalpesh Abhani, Mr Nilesh Hapani, Mr Hasit Hadani, Mr Hardik Trivedi, Mr Chetan Sangani, Mr Chirag Maseta and Mr Devendra Bansode deserve a warm thanks. I thank my teachers Dr Bharti Bais, Drs (Mr and Mrs) Taji and Dr Pranjal Sharma from the deapth of my heart.

I am thankful to Dr K Park, who is one of the best authors in the field of preventive and social medicine, for providing me with the statistical and numerical references for this book. I thank my work place – Max New York life insurance Company – where I served and learnt the practical perspective of weight management in the insurance sector. My sincere thanks to my, the then colleagues and seniors working with me, Mrs Nina Vyas, Mr Ajay Patil and Ms Shipla Mangala, Mr Sanjiv Pathank, Dr Nootan Ghosh and Dr Nitin Gupta – for providing me with the insight for practical application of obesity in determining quality of life. I thank the learning which was imparted to me through the discussions with Mr Gurmit Singh, Mrs Madhavi Munshi and Mrs Punita Sharma Arora of Advance Therapeutics and Mr Amit Bohora, Dr Pedro of Biosensors – in my careers course was a great motivation behind completion of this work.

Last but not the least, my sincere thanks to the Directors and staff of B Jain publishers and to all who have directly and indirectly helped in the making of this book – deserve the greatest thanks with a wide smile.

Publisher's Note

The visually disproportionate fatty growth in the physical appearance of an individual definitely impacts his life and personality in a major way. The chubby looks, the distended abdomen, fat look on face, handles on sides of the tummy – are all things that definitely do not give a pleasant appearance to the people around. All these are the different signs of obesity which this book discusses; and also gives the 50 things that cause so much inconsistency to the body parts. Obesity, which happens, mainly due to the uneven distribution of fat on the various areas of the body can be controlled in a major way.

This is an effort by the Health and Harmony team of B Jain publishers to reach to the masses with the objective to educate them to find better treatment for themselves.

B Jain publishers are serving the society with health books for the past five decades, imparting knowledge gathered by different well-known doctors of the era. It is very important for an individual to know his body well to have a healthy future.

Kuldeep Jain
C.E.O., B. Jain Publishers (P) Ltd.

Contents

Preface .... *iii*

Acknowledgements .... *v*

Publisher's Note .... *vii*

CHAPTERS

1. Obesity: General Considerations 1
2. Physiology of Fat and Causes of Obesity 35
3. Metabolic Causes of Obesity 53
4. Obesity and underlying Diseases 81
5. Treatment of Obesity: Diet and Exercise 129
6. Treatment of Obesity: Medication and Counselling 177
7. Complications of Obesity 189
8. 50 Don'ts of Obesity: The Way to Avoid Obesity and its Related Complications 199

9.	Apendix I – Conditions Including Obesity, Overweight and Weight Gain	215
	Apendix II – Fat Burners	221
	Apendix III – Calorie Content of Common Food Material	226

Chapter 1

Obesity: General Considerations

Many of us today have various concepts about obesity. Apart from the cosmetic perspective, there is a growing awareness about its effect on health, be it the level of activeness or the risk of various diseases, any which way, it makes an impact on our personality. Most of us always want to be fit and fine, have a good figure and good body statistics. In spite of all the facts just quoted, obesity is the fastest growing non-communicable health condition. Almost one third of young American population and almost half the adults are overweight. A similar scenario is present in India and a graver one in Europe. This is what makes me concerned and drives to write something that may help save a chubby burden on world's health budget. There are various indicators of obesity and its related risks. Relationship of obesity with nutrition is also relooked and explored better in recent days. Many healthcare organisations have taken obesity into their primary care agenda. Although many efforts are being made, regular focus in most cases is more or less on the cosmetic perspective. Many obese subjects, indifferent to their physical appearance are less educated about the risks of obesity on their health. Additionally, there are various social aspects of overfeeding in human beings, one of the most common causes of obesity in developing countries.

Recently published studies and statistics have demonstrated obesity as having a direct relation with cardiac and some metabolic conditions. Still, in spite of several considerations connotations and theories born out of gravid research, many whims and fancies about obesity are flickering around as "medical myths".

What is Obesity?

Obesity is a relative term which is defined by many systems by their own customised definitions. The factors which we use commonly to define obesity are pertaining to the physical appearance. More or less, visually disproportionate fatty growth is labeled as obesity in day-to-day practice. Chubby looks, distended abdomen, fat look of face, presence of love handles on the sides of tummy, broad waist, broad trunk, etc. are considered as signs of obesity. All the listed parameters reflect, again, the cosmetic concerns about obesity and in about seven cases out of ten, these are indeed perfect. Every tenth case of obesity may be missed from diagnosis due to various reasons, if only these parameters are followed.

Consideration of weight alone may not be diagnostic enough. Weight of an individual depends upon various factors. Considering the weight and height or the body mass index, makes an all-inclusive definition of obesity in non-body-builders. Per se, obesity or an overweight body is a disproportionate increase of body especially due to excess of non-muscular body mass. There are various indices and numerical definitions designed for obesity. The most commonly followed is Body Mass Index (BMI), according to which, a body mass index of more than 25 is clearly considered as obesity. This definition does not apply to body builders. Myotoned bodies need to be evaluated by the hip to waist ratio and the shoulder to tummy height ratio.

By medical definition, *'Obesity is an abnormal growth of body's adipose (fat) tissue due to increase in size or number or both of the fat cells'*. Medical statistic standard of obesity is a body mass index more than 30 in males and 28 in females.*

Obesity, as already discussed is not necessarily meaning a chubby tummy. In almost three cases out of ten, it may not be present, even in subjects defined as obese by medical science. This may happen due to the distribution of fat on various areas of the body, or almost on all body parts. For understanding this better, we need to understand the types of obesity and pattern of fat distribution in the body.

Types of Obesity

There are a few patterns of fat distribution in the body. There are some areas where fat is always deposited in even non-obese subjects. The fat deposition patterns in males and females differ pertaining to the hormones particular to their reproductive system. In fact, this makes a first differentiation of fat distribution patterns; whether healthy or obese. In case of obesity, the other pattern of fat distribution is more concerning. Depending upon this distribution of fat deposition in various body parts, obesity is divisible as central obesity and general obesity.

---

*(Refer – Park's *Text book of Preventive and Social Medicine,* edition XXV).

Central Obesity

Central obesity refers to deposition of adipose tissue on and about the central axis. The fat is mostly seen over the abdominal belly, chest especially the pectoral region, buttocks, frontal neck and lower face. The adiposity is less in arms, thighs, back, legs, etc. Formation of a bulky abdomen, love handles, buffalo hump and gynecomastia is commonly seen in this pattern of adiposity. Most of the hormonal conditions such as, Cushing's Syndrome commonly display this pattern of adiposity.

This obesity is of the most common type and is seen in most parts of the world. About 70 percent of all obesity cases are of this type. This obesity is common in elderly people yet can be seen in young subjects also. Sometimes, this type of obesity is seen in sedentary workers, despite a body mass index within normal range.

General Obesity

General obesity is where fat deposition is more or less even in most of the body parts. From this, we do not mean disproportionate growth of leaner organs like hands, but the fat distribution is uniformly proportionate to the part's size. The fat is deposited on the abdominal belly, pectorals, buttocks, back, nape and front of neck, shoulders, arms and thighs. In this pattern, the body looks stout, broad chested, especially in earlier days. This pattern (general obesity) is observed commonly in young ages and in those who had heavy physical stress in previous days. The obesity related to nutritional deficiencies is also one of the commonest causes of this pattern. This obesity is observed to be slower in development and progress.

There are some patterns specific to certain geographic areas. Middle East shows a common pattern of obesity called Middle East pattern. This pattern pertains to their customary food habits such as excess of eating beef. In this pattern, the fat is particularly more on the belly and back, below the skin of all joints and at the nape of the neck.

Western pattern of adiposity is a type of general obesity which is more severe and bulkier around the trunk and heighted belly. Usually this pattern is associated with thin legs and tapering thighs. Similar features are there in arms and forearms but less severe.

Depending upon the tendency to adiposity, the body's shape is also determined. Subjects tending to retain adiposity at hips and buttocks are called pear bodied, while people who are fat mostly in the abdomen have an apple body shape.

Indices of Obesity

Many times, even now, the primary assessment of obesity is by visual perception. Though visual perception gives information regarding one's physical structure, some facts and measurements are required for the actual establishment of diagnosis, and risk calculations. For this practical purpose, a few anthropometric norms have been evolved. Relative and comparative assessment of these measurement data points form a good source as index for obesity and related risks.

Anthropometry for Assessment of Obesity

1. Girths (Circumference)

They are measured with wrapping a tailor's tape around the desired organ. These measurements are written in inches as well as in centimeters. The subject is usually in standing position for this measurement.

a. Abdomen: Highest abdominal circumference.

b. Chest (Unexpanded): This is measured across the nipples.

c. Hips: Measured across both hip joints.

d. Waist: Measured across the highest points on bony prominences on both sides of the abdomen – this is a tailor's measurement for stitching your clothes.

e. Arm: Measured at the mid of the arm.

f. Thigh: Measured at the mid of the thigh.

g. Calf: Measured at the highest point, below the knee.

h. Neck: Measured at any point between the jaw and the base of the neck.

2. Height

It is measured in various positions, which make them anatomically and meteorologically significant. All heights are noted at their highest points.

a. Standing height of body without shoes.

b. Lying abdominal belly height.

c. Lying shoulder height.

d. Lying knee height.

3. Weight

Weight of a person is measured in a standing weighing scale, without shoes and preferably without clothes. However, in routine the weight is always taken with clothes, hence, the type of clothes worn should at least be standardised. The weight is noted in pounds as well as in kilograms. All indices of obesity consider weight in kilograms.

Weight disproportionate to height is the commonest index of obesity, especially in adults. Rather, most of the people assess their current weight statistics considering the weight they have been comfortably living with, in the close past. This happens but with figure-conscious or weight conscious people. There are height-weight charts as follows for consideration of men and women. Table 1.1 has standard height and weight combinations for the average population. This is a standard chart for Asian and European population. Standard weight + 5 is for Americans, and standard weight + 3 for the African population in reference to this chart.

Table 1.1 Metropolitan Weight Chart

Height	Men			Women		
Meters	Desirable Average	Desirable Weight Range	Obese	Desirable Average	Desirable Weight Range	Obese
1.45				46.0	42-53	64
1.48				46.5	42-54	65
1.5				47.0	43-55	66
1.52				48.5	44-57	68
1.54				49.5	44-58	70
1.56				50.4	45-58	70
1.58	55.8	51-64	77	51.3	56-59	71
1.6	57.6	52-65	78	52.6	48-61	73
1.62	58.6	53-66	79	54.0	49-62	74
1.64	59.6	54-67	80	55.4	50-64	77
1.66	60.6	55-69	83	56.8	51-65	78
1.68	61.7	56-71	85	58.1	52-66	79
1.7	63.5	58-73	88	60.0	53-67	80
1.72	65	59-74	89	61.30	55-69	83
1.74	66.5	60-75	90	62.60	56-70	84
1.76	68	62-77	92	64.00	58-72	86
1.78	69.4	64-79	95	65.30	50-74	89
1.8	71	65-80	96			
1.82	72.6	66-82	98			
1.84	74.2	67-84	101			
1.86	75.8	69-86	103			
1.88	77.6	71-88	106			
1.9	79.3	73-90	108			
1.92	81	75-93	112			

Indices with Mathematical Calculations

Indices derived from anthropometric data by mathematical calculations are relatively better indices for obesity and its related risks. These calculations take input from the measurements, process the data with certain formula(e) and provide competitive outputs. As these indices form a relative standard, they are applicable universally. For example, body mass index (BMI) is calculation of weight per body's surface area; this relates height with the weight. Considering the fact that a particular weight may be more for a person with some height, the same may be normal or low for a person with some other height. The body mass index gives a more specific idea. There are several calculations and standardisations in all these indices, which we will consider further.

These indices are:

1. Broca's index
2. Lorentz formula
3. Body mass index
4. Poderal index
5. Waist to hip ratio
6. Saggital abdominal diameter (Lying belly height)
7. Shoulder to belly ratio

8. Skin fold thickness
9. Body fat percentage

1. Broca's index

Broca's index is a simple calculation based on the person's height, to determine the median weight. This formula gives a desirable approximate weight. This usually has a variation from metropolitan weight chart and has more of an American trend in it. The cutoff point for obesity is taken as Median height + 2 bands further.

W_{avg} = Height of the person in cm (H) – 100

For example, if a person has a height of 164 cm (5'6"), the desired average weight will be 64 kg. The cutoff limit for obesity will be at 70 kg (standard at band of 170 cm or 5'8" height).

This formula is widely used for common calculations but has limitations while demonstrating risk profile. Also, as the standard weight calculation may differ in males and females, this forms another limitation to the formula.

2. Lorentz formula

This is more specific than Broca's index. This makes the Broca's index more specific in general population of all types. This formula removes the error of male and female average weight, and median weight taint.

The formula is:

D_{Women} = (height in cm (H) – 100) – [(height in cm (H)–150) / 2] kg

D_{Men} = (height in cm – 100) – [(height in cm–150)/ 4] kg

For example, for a woman of height (H) 160 cm, the standard weight D is:

$$D = (160 - 100) - [(160 - 150)/2]$$
$$= 60 - [10/2]$$
$$= 55 \text{ kg}$$

Average weight (D) calculated from this formula is closely similar to the average weight described in metropolitan weight chart. The cutoff for obesity is set at + 2 bands from the average desired weight.

3. Body mass index

Body mass index or BMI is a more sensitive and standard index for obesity. All calculations, risk ratios, statistics and prevalence or demographics and health assessments, are based upon BMI. BMI virtually refers to the weight per square meter of body surface area. It is easier for calculation and simpler for understanding. In medical statistics and according to WHO recommendations, BMI has a unique stature. It is calculated in the following manner:

BMI = Weight in kg/Square of height in m

For example, if your height is 167 cm and weight is 70 kgs; that is, the height in meters is 1.67 meters, a square of this is 2.7889 = 2.89

BMI = 70 / 2.89 is 24.22 ≈ 24

Let us take another system of measures. Suppose the height is 5 feet and 7 inches, conversion factor is approximately 2.54 cm = 1 inch.

Thus, 5' 7" = 67" = 67 x 2.54 = 170.18 cm = 1.7 m.

Suppose weight is 63 kg.

Now BMI is 63/2.89 = 21.7 ≈ 22

In the third example, take the weight as 120 lbs (pounds) and height as 5' 2".

Height in meters will be 1.57 and weight – 120 / 2.2 = 54.54 kg

Thus BMI is 22.1 ≈ 22

An ideal BMI is between 19 and 23. BMI more than 24 but less than 28 is in some opinions borderline overweight but not obese. In females, a BMI more than 28 and in males, a BMI more than 30 is clearly obesity. For children, the BMI is ideal from 17 to 22 as they grow rapidly. Hence, there the BMI alone is not enough to evaluate the obesity status. The risk of cardiac diseases, metabolic diseases, etc. increase with every unit of increase in BMI. Also, when BMI is calculated in the metric system, the standard banding deviations are compact. The errors of calculation due to standardisation errors are also eliminated.

There are alternative formulae for imperial system calculations of BMI but they are less popular.

BMI = Weight in pounds x 4.88 / height in feet^2

Or

Weight in pounds x 703 / height in inches^2

4. Ponderal index

This index is calculated in reciprocate manner to the BMI. The index has more specificity in cases where BMI information needs to be revalidated. This is virtual interrelation linear weight distribution or in other words, density of the body. Ponderal index is not very popular due to the difficult mathematical calculations. This method is less common but has higher validity especially in very short stature. Practical implementation of this method is not easy in its basic form as the parameter is not statistically stratified easily. Hence, the formula has many expressions:

PI = (Height in centimeters / cube root of body weight in kgs)

For example, person's height is 164 cm, w 64 kg,

PI = 164 / 4 = 41

Other Expressions of Ponderal Index

Table 1.2 Expressions of Ponderal Index

Formula	Range
PI= Weight in kg / Height in Meters^3	Adults – 10.3 to 13.9
	Infants – 24
PI = 100* x Cube root of weight in kg/ Height in cm	2.175 to 2.4

Body health is not influenced by quantity of body fat alone. In fact, location-wise distribution of the fat is also equally important. Based upon the fat distribution pattern, as discussed previously, the body can be analogues to a pear shape or an apple shape. Subjects tending to retain adiposity at hips and buttocks are called pear bodied, while people who have fat mostly in the abdomen have an apple body shape.

Apple shaped body group of people, have increased risk for morbidity linked to obesity than pear shaped body group of people. Hence for this, evaluation of fat distribution pattern is also very important. The indices of obesity that work on the basis of anthropometric comparison method, have features for assessing fat distribution.

5. Waist to Hip Ratio

Waist to hip ratio is not an index of obesity per se, but is one of the most sensitive indices for morbidity (disease causing nature) related to obesity. As known, obesity may be a direct risk factor for heart disease. This has been proven by research in recent days. The lying belly height or standing waist to hip ratio is a sensitive measurement for this purpose. For this ratio, both the measurements are taken in inches.

Method for measurement of Waist to Hip Ratio

a. Measurement of the Hip: The hip is measured at the highest part on it, across the buttocks. Ilium is a bony prominence felt on the sides in front of the waist. Just below these bony prominences, the hip region starts. The circumference is measured with a tailor's tape.

Abdominal Belly Circumference (Waist): The abdominal belly height is measured for the maximum, by sliding a circumflexed tape over the belly from below the chest to the waist in a standing position. The highest measurement is taken for calculation.

b. Calculation of the Ratio:

$R = (H_{max}/B_{max})$ where B_{Max} is the maximum belly circumference (waist)

H_{max} is maximum hip circumference

and R is the risk ratio

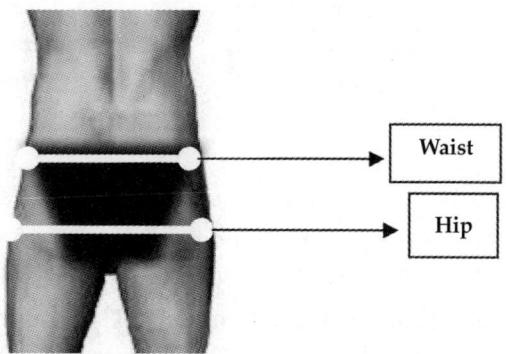

Fig. 1.1 Measurement of Waist to Hip

For example, if the belly circumference is 32" and the hip is 30", the risk ratio is 0.9.

Table 1.3 Ratio Interpretation

Health risk based solely on WHR	Male	Female
Safe	< 0.8	< .65
Borderline	0.81 - 0.89	0.66 - 0.74
Low risk	0.90 - 0.95	0.75 - 0.80
Moderate risk	0.96 - 1.0	0.81 - 0.85
High risk	> 1.0	> 0.85
Alarming	> 1.05	> 0.95

The hip to waist ratio is also considered as a measurement of beauty for body, especially in women. 36-24-36 is the commonest measurement code for hip – waist – chest.

Factors to be Considered

i. *Age:* With growing age this ratio tends to be a bit higher. Hence, a relatively higher ratio with regular BMI may be considered fine but needs to be monitored regularly.

ii. *Sex:* Women before menopause may have a different ratio, and they are known to have higher cardiac disease risk. The waist to hip ratio in this age group may be a bit high, but must be critically evaluated.

iii. *Pregnancy:* This should be excluded in calculation of risk ratio.

iv. *Known Ascites:* Protein energy malnutrition need to be excluded.

6. Abdominal Height in Lying Down Position

This measurement is also called supine abdominal diameter or supine abdominal height. Lying abdominal height is considered and demonstrated to be a better index for obesity related diseases especially the cardiac conditions. Higher abdominal belly height is highly related to the risk of cardiac illness. Studies in recent days have successfully co-related belly height to risk of cardiac illness. A Cohort study (published in the American Journal of Epidemiology, where 101,765 patents were evaluated from 1965 to 70; the follow up was taken after 12 years) has shown higher mortality in high abdominal belly people. From this study, the supine abdominal diameter is considered a sensitive index of obesity related risk, separately of BMI. This index for visceral fat is more predictive of the risk. Almost all patients having abdominal obesity are prone to have cardiovascular diseases. Approximately one third have a risk of cancers and one fifth have a risk to metabolic conditions. More than half the subjects of this type carry a predisposition to diabetes.

Method of Measurement

Subject should be in lying down position. A flat plane subject such as a notebook should be held at the highest point on the belly, parallel to the plan of supination. The height between these two planes is noted in centimeters and inches. This height is abdominal belly diameter in supine position. The diameter in adults should be less than 20 cm. 20–25 cm is borderline and more than 25 cm is definitely high. For clinical research purposes, this evaluation is done at the level of iliac spine with a sliding beam calipers.

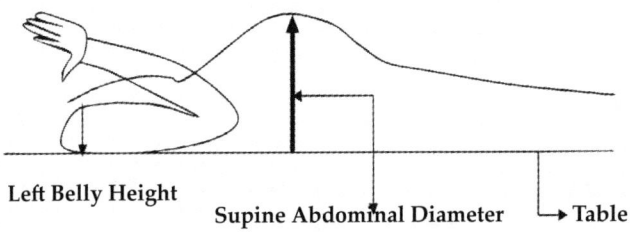

Fig. 1.2 Method of Measurement

Evaluation

As per the studied standards, the evaluation of abdominal height (sagittal abdominal diameter) is itself the most sensitive parameter of obesity related to cardiac risk. Any abdominal height more than 25 cm is at the risk of cardiac diseases and diabetes and most of the population with an abdominal height of more than 28 cm develops hypertension very early in life.

7. Shoulder to Belly Ratio

It is also one of the indices but it has a limited accountability.

i. Abdomen height / Shoulder height < 1. good

ii. Abdominal height / Shoulder height > 1.2 risk increases with increasing ratio

8. Skin Fold Thickness

Most common storage area for the fat is the tissue below the skin. There is a lot of adipose tissue under the skin, which forms the thickness of the skin. Skin fold thickness is a very clear indicator of deposition of adipose tissue under the skin. Higher the skin fold thickness, higher is the fat deposition. Usually, the output of the final calculation of the method is the percentage of body fat. This determines the body's fat composition and hence the aging of the body. There are several methods developed for measuring skin fold thickness. This itself reveals its inevitable importance.

Measurement of Skin Fold Thickness

Skin fold thickness is measured by several methods. The most commonly used two methods are physical and X-ray absorptiometry. Other methods like bioelectrical methods are less popular now.

Areas for Skin Fold Thickness Measurement

A fold of skin from specific areas is taken for measurement of skin fold thickness. These areas are those where a proper double fold of skin of enough height can be taken with adipose tissue. There are five such areas in the anterior of the body and two such in the posterior.

Areas in the anterior region are:

a. *Chest:* Draw a line between the nipple and the armpit. A pinch of skin fold in the same direction is taken for measurement. In men, this is at the midpoint of this line, and in women, the point at the armpit side, one-third of this line is chosen.

b. *Middle of the Armpit:* A vertical fold can be taken on a line running down the armpit, called the mid-axillary line.

c. *Abdomen:* A little tilted vertical pinch besides the navel on the belly can be taken for measurement. A diagonal fold on the side of the abdomen, where there is a bony prominence can also be used for measurement. Ideally, the skin-folds for measurement in abdomen is pinched one inch above the bony prominence of pelvis in all these three locations.

d. *Thigh:* A vertical fold of skin on the thigh, on the midline of thigh at the midpoint between the knee and hip can be taken.

Areas in the posterior region are:

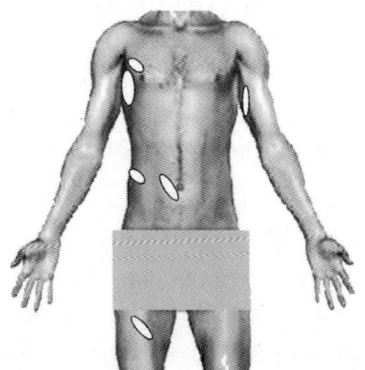

Fig. 1.3 Areas of the Posterior Region

a. *Behind the arm* (triceps area).

b. *On the blades of shoulder joint* – the scapular area.

All these areas have vertical folds.

Method 1 – Physical Measurement

For physical measurement, skinfold thickness calipers are required. These calipers from various makers are available in the market. Alternatively, blunt forceps and a scale can be used but this is comparatively vague.

Method for Measurement

Skinfold measurement is taken in standing position. When we feel between the index finger and thumb, we can feel in most cases, two layers, one shallow and another deep. We have to take the pinch deep enough, so that it includes the fat layer. Do not bother if a muscle gets pulled in the pinch, in all these areas, muscles are tight and deep enough. Also, we are following such direction, where pulling in of muscles is impossible.

Now measure the thickness of this fold, either by a pair of calipers, or by placing a forceps and measuring the gap within the arms of the forceps. Three such readings are taken and averaged for each fold. This will minimise the human and mechanical error. The skin fold thickness should be less than 15 mm for a good fat profile.

9. Estimation of Body's Fat Percentage

There are several methods for calculating body's fat content (percentage). The most used and reliable method is hydrolic density evaluation. Other methods are considerably good in performance, yet they have limits.

a. From skin fold thickness – Bone density

b. From BMI and body girths

a. Skin Fold Thickness – Bone Density

For calculation of body fat from skinfold method, seven (all of above) fords or three folds (pectoral, lateral abdominal and thigh) are taken into consideration. All these measurements are taken in millimeters.

Prerequisites

Age of the subject, sex, height, weight (latter two for calculation of BMI), bone marrow density.

The format for body fat percentage is:

% BF= [(4.95/Bone density) - 4.5] x 100

This formula is called SIRI formula.

There is an alternative formula called Brozek formula:

% BF = (4.57/Bone marrow density − 4.142) × 100

The SIRI formula is more accepted.

Calculation of Bone Marrow Density

Seven folds measured —

BMD Women = [1.097 - (0.00046971 x Sum 7)] + (0.00000056 x Sum 7^2) − (0.00012828 x Age)

BMD Men = 1.1093800 - (0.0008267 x Sum 7) + (0.0000056 x Sum 7^2) − (0.0002574 x Age)

Three folds measured —

BMD = 1.0994921 - (0.0009929 x Sum 3) + (0.0000023 x Sum 3^2) - (0.0001392 x Age)

For example,

Parameter	Value
Age	32
Sex	Female
Height	153
Weight	59
BMI	**25.20398137**

Skin Fold Area	Thickness in mm
Pectoral	15
Mid-axillary	12
Suprailiac (Lateral Abdominal)	18
Abdominal	15
Thigh	10
On the Shoulder Blade Apex	8
Back of the Arm	7

BMD	**1.05701569**
%BF =	**18.29957652**

Alternately, the three fold method can also be used. For example,

Parameter	Value
Age	32
Sex	Male
Height	153
Weight	59
BMI	**23.030045**

Skin Fold Area	Thickness in mm
Pectoral	15
Mid-axillary	—
Suprailiac (Lateral Abdominal)	18
Abdominal	—
Thigh	10
On the Shoulder Blade Apex	—
Back of the Arm	—
	43
Bone Density	**1.056596**
% Body Fat	**18.48572**

Method 2

This method is automatic with the X-ray beam absorbometry device. Then, the bone density and body fat percentage is calculated mathematically.

b. Calculation of Body Fat Percentage from BMI

BMI is also used to calculate body fat percentage,

Prerequisites:

Height, weight, age of the person.

Formulae

- Body Fat % $_{Child\ male}$ = (1.51 x BMI) - (0.70 x Age) - (3.6 x 1) + 1.4
- Body Fat % $_{Child\ female}$ = (1.51 x BMI) - (0.70 x Age) - (3.6 x 0) + 1.4
- Body Fat % $_{Adult\ male}$ = (1.20 x BMI) + (0.23 x Age) - (10.8 x 1) - 5.4
- Body Fat % $_{Adult\ female}$ = (1.20 x BMI) + (0.23 x Age) - (10.8 x 0) - 5.4

For example,

Parameter	Value
Age	35
Sex	Male
Height	168
Weight	64
BMI	**22.675737**
Body Fat %	**19.060884**

US navy method of calculation of body fat percentage from various body measurements, but this method is not very accurate:

For Men:

a. 86.010*LOG (Abdomen – Neck $^{\text{in inches}}$) - 70.041*LOG (Height $^{\text{in inches}}$) + 36.7

b. 86.010*LOG (Abdomen–Neck $^{\text{in centimeters}}$) - 70.041*LOG (Height $^{\text{in centimeters}}$) + 30.30

For Women:

a. 163.205*LOG (Abdomen + Hip – Neck $^{\text{in inches}}$) - 97.684*LOG (Height $^{\text{in inches}}$) - 78.387

b. 163.205*LOG (Abdomen + Hip - Neck $^{\text{in centimeters}}$) - 97.684*LOG (Height $^{\text{in centimeters}}$) - 104.912

For example,

Neck	26
Abdomen	80
Height	168
Sex	Male
%BF	**23.44**

Evaluation of Body Fat Percentage

Description	Women	Men
Essential Fat (Minimum)	10–13	2-5
Athletic Body	14–20	6-13
Fit Body – Active – Non-athletic	21–24	14–17
Healthy – Acceptable (Sedentary)	25–31	18–24
Obese	32 +	25 +

Absolute Excess Fat and Minimum Excess Fat

Absolute and minimum excess fat is calculated in the following steps:

A1 – Calculated body fat % – Essential body fat % = Absolute excess fat %

A2 – Calculated body fat % – Average body fat % in your body type = Absolute excess fat %

B – Weight x A 1 = Absolute body fat , Weight x A2 = Minimum body fat

For example,

Parameter	Value
Age	32
Sex	Male
Height	168
Weight	65
% Body Fat	18.48572

(A1) Absolute excess body fat % man = 18.5 – 3 (Average between 2-5) = 15.5%

(A2) Minimum excess body fat % man, sedentary = 18.5 – 21 (Average between 18 – 24) = – 2.5%

From the above, absolute body fat of this person is calculated as 15.5% x 65 kg that equals to 10.1 kg. This means if a person has to lose weight, 10.1 kg fat from the body should be lost by consumption. In this case, there is no need for weight loss as the BMI and the body fat percentage is within the range of non-obesity. If at all some fat burning exercise is started, the person will become more active and get a fitter body.

In this capter, we have discussed all important points of obesity in general. We now understand the various concepts and misconcepts about obesity. This chapter helps to evaluate where we stand with our body type considering fat distribution and obesity. Further more, we understand how our body deals with fats, how useful and harmful the fats are for us, how does one become obese and how to deal or treat obesity.

Review and Recap

1. Obesity is abnormal growth of body's adipose (fat) tissue due to increase in size or number or both of fat cells.

2. Though visual perception gives information of one's physical structure, some facts and measurements are required for the actual establishment of diagnosis and risk calculations. For this practical purpose, a few anthropometric norms have been evolved. Relative and comparative assessment of these measurement data forms a good source as an index for obesity and its related risks.

3. Weight disproportionate to height is the commonest index of obesity, especially in adults.

4. As a particular weight may be more for a person with a particular height, the same may be normal or low for a person having a different height or some other both type, body mass index or BMI gives a more specific idea. But BMI does not consider fat distribution.

5. Ideal BMI is between 19 and 23. BMI more than 24 but less than 28 is in some opinions borderline overweight but not obese. In females, BMI more than 28 and in males, BMI more than 30 is clearly obesity. For children, BMI is ideal from 17 to 22.
6. High risk waist to hip ratio is > 1.0 in males and > 0.85 in females.
7. Any abdominal height more than 25 cm is at risk of cardiac disease and diabetes, and most of the population with an abdominal height of more than 28 develops hypertension at a very early stage.
8. Absolute body fat means the amount of fat that should be burnt from body for weight loss. This is calculated by subtracting permissible range of fat for your body type from total fat percentage currently your body has. This amount is considered minimum losable fat in the body by calculations but this will be the maximum (Upper limit) amount of fat to be lost when you are losing weight. If a person in acceptable fat range starts fat burning exercises, the person will become more active and get a fitter body. Practically, this should be the basis of diet modification.

Chapter 2
Physiology of Fat and Causes of Obesity

We now already know many things about body's adiposity (obesity). We have already understood fat deposition and methods to understand its distribution and evaluation. Now, before we proceed into further details regarding obesity in general, let us discuss the body's physiology of fat metabolism and some pathophysiology of obesity. This will help us in understanding obesity or fat deposition in the body in a wider and more scientific perspective.

Fat Metabolism of the Body

Like all other food articles, fat is taken in the body along with ingested food. Fat ingestion in the body is followed by its digestion, absorption and metabolism.

Some amount of fat is created in the body itself by conversion of excessive glucose into fat material. Fat is a storable source of energy in the body, that can be stored for long periods of time. With growing age, this store goes on increasing. In other words, fat storage in the body determines the aging of the body. There are specific areas in the body prone to retain fats. These areas vary in the male and female body, though there are certain common areas also. The purpose of storing of fat in common areas is specific.

Common compounds labeled as fat in the body are:

1. Neutral fats or triglycerides
2. Phospholipids
3. Cholesterol

There are various other less significant fat compounds which may be present in smaller quantities that have a fat label on them besides these three. In a nutshell, all compounds which have a chemistry of fatty acids will be taken in this group.

Sources of Fat in the Body

There are two types of sources of the fat in the body, which are as follows.

1. The first, being ingested as a part of food. It contributes the maximum fat in our body.
2. The second part is the fat anabolised in the body by conversion of excess glucose and all fructose to triglycerides.

The most important part is to understand various phenomena taking place to create, maintain and consume the fat source in the body.

Intake of Fat

Just like all other nutrients, the major source of fat intake is ingestion with food. This intake is mainly two parts. The first part is sensible fats - direct intake of fats from animal and vegetable sources like butter, ghee, oils and animal fats. Non-sensible intake of fat comprises of volatile and essential oils from vegetables, grains, flesh etc. volatile and essential oils in vegetables and grains are the main source of fat in the food. All this fat is digested and absorbed in the intestines. In a typical balanced meal, approximately 5 percent of the total food should be fats. This should constitute approximately 25 grams and 225 Cal/Calories energy for a 65 kg body with 170 cm height.

Digestion of Fat

Fat is digested in the intestines. Various enzymes from the liver and intestines are responsible for digestion of fat. Fat is converted into small particles called Chylomicrons. Chylomicrons are basically large fatty acid particles. These fatty acids are formed as a result of the action of intestinal contents on the fat ingested and fragmented into small particles by the stomach and intestinal movements.

Absorption and Transport

Chylomicrons are absorbed in the small intestines and are released into the lymphatics. Some proteins, released simultaneously with fats, combine with chylomicrons and form absorb. This absorb enters the blood stream in routine course with the lymph. Approximately, two hours after a fat rich diet, plasma concentration of chylomicrons rises by 1-2 per cent. This gives plasma a turbid yellow look. It is but cleared from blood very rapidly.

Synthesis of Fat in the Body

Lipogenesis is the process by which fat cells store fat as triglycerides. This happens in the adipocytes.

Inner fatty acids are synthesised by the liver. The source of this is majorly carbohydrates and minor proteins. All fructose that is ingested is converted into fat, especially triglycerides. Any glucose in excess amount is also stored as fats. Free fatty acids, generated as a result of digestion, enter the circulation. These fatty acids are then metabolised into triglycerides, very low density lipoproteins (VLDL), and released into the circulation.

Some fatty acids (either from digestion or as a result of breaking down of triglycerides) are imbibed by the adipocytes. These fatty acids imbibed in the adipocytes are again converted to triglycerides and than stored into triglycerides in store.

Clearance of Fat from Blood

Fat clearance from blood occurs in liver and adipose tissue. When blood passes through these two areas, the chylomicrons adsorbs are removed from blood and are stored in the area temporarily. The fat clearance from blood occurs with 6-12 hours in usual cases. And after a meal, the plasma fat levels return to baseline after this.

Breaking of Triglycerides – Lipolysis

Lipolysis means generating free fatty acids. This may happen for two reasons:

1. For energy utilisation within the body.
2. For reformation into triglycerides within the adipocyte as stated above.

Lipolysis within the adipocyte is influenced by lipase enzyme. This enzyme is actually called hormone sensitive lipase. Hormone sensitive lipase can be acted and activated by hormones of the Suprarenal glands such as epinephrine (adrenalin), nor-epinephrine (nor-adrenalin), corticotrophin and glucocorticoids. Other hormones such as growth hormone, thyroid hormone and insulin have an important role or influence the activation of this lipase.

Storage of Fats

Lipogenesis and lipolysis take place within the adipocyte. Excess of free triglycerides are lipolised along with digestive fatty acids and are taken into the adipose tissue. In this tissue or in the liver, these fatty acids are re-synthesised as storable triglyceride material and are stored there in the respective (adipose / liver) tissues. The major storage of fat is in adipose tissues. Common areas where fat is stored are as follows.

1. Some important artery beds (stable) like coronary artery
2. Buttocks (increasing)
3. Abdominal muscles (increasing)
4. Mesentery (stable)
5. Palms, soles (stable)
6. Under the skin (increasing)

Based upon the storage of fat in the body areas, patterns are formed which have been discussed in the earlier chapter.

Storage of fats is also influenced by some hormones. Estrogen, corticosteroids and growth hormone lead to storage of fats whereas thyroxin and up to an extent, insulin release fat from these stores for utilisation. As most steroidal hormones are gonad related, the patterns of male and female bodies in relation to fat deposition show specific patterns.

Specific fat storage areas in men:

1. Abdomen, especially the sides (love handles) and the belly.
2. Some skeletal areas such as back, neck, arms and thighs.

Specific fat storage areas in women:

1. Buttocks and glutei region muscles
2. Loins and lower back
3. Breasts
4. Thighs

Females, under the influence of estrogen, have excessive fat storage in the body, as compared to the males. These fats also bring a specific feminine shape to their body. In fact, such fat storage is a type of boon; they are less subject to diseases from cholesterol deposition.

Utility of Fats in the Body

1. As a stored energy.
2. Binding and modifying proteins for various building activity (like lipoproteins).
3. Making a thick padding for protection of delicate internal organs.

Hormone Effect

Insulin and catecholamines (adrenalin and non-adrenalin) influence fat metabolism the most.

Catecholamines are main stimulants of lipolysis. Release of catecholamines like adrenalin and nor adrenalin increase metabolism in the body as a response to increased requirements. Increased body metabolism with consequent requirements for energy. Catecholamine act through two channels, α (alpha) and β (beta) receptor channel. β receptors promote lipolysis and predominate. In conditions associated with greater fat deposition such as fasting, diabetes mellitus, hypothyroidism, pregnancy, the predominance is shifted to α receptors.

Insulin promotes lipogenesis, inhibits lipolysis, and stimulates hepatic gluconeogenesis. It is one form which activates lipoprotein lipase and facilitates glucose transport into the adipocytes. After glucose is stored in the body, insulin promotes its conversion into fats and triglycerides. Other mediators of lipolysis include adreno-corticotropic hormone (ACTH), which stimulates the secretion of suprarenal corticoids, thyroid stimulating hormone (TSH), by releasing thyroid hormones, growth hormone and vasopressin (ADH).

Growth hormone and thyroid hormone act almost opposite to each other. Thyroid hormones increase consumption of fat for release of energy and conserve glucose. Growth hormone acts in the converse way.

Pathophysiology of Obesity

Balance between intake of energy in the form of food and utilisation of energy in bodily activities is based upon feed-back mechanism of requirements. An enzyme called leptin produces nerve signals for satiety and hunger based upon positive or negative feedback of energy requirements. Depending upon one's requirement of the body, as discussed earlier, a "weight set point" for an individual person is determined by his or her body requirements and eating habits. This "weight set point" eventually get reset when there is a sustained modification of diet and exercise pattern in certain circumstances. Considering all these points, several laws of thermodynamics are used to explain the pathophysiology of obesity. Although this is a multifactorial phenomenon and has many etiological considerations, these few parts are common to all.

'Obesity results when there is an imbalance between energy expenditure and energy intake.'

The Energy Expenditure

1. *Utilisation of energy in the body to maintain metabolism and basal metabolic rate (BMR):*

   This can be considered as resting energy consumption. The body's resting active actions such as heart and lung, gastrointestinal tract function and passive activity such as kidney, liver and brain functions also consume some energy. Also, some amount of metabolic heat is always generated in the body to maintain a basic body temperature. This whole energy expenditure is called 'basal metabolism' and the energy consumed to maintain the basal metabolic rate is 'basal energy expenditure.'

There are several factors which affect the basal metabolism of a person. The major factor that influences this part is body mass excluding fat. In other words, higher the amount of muscle, more is the basal metabolic rate. Thyroid hormones, especially thyroxin is very influential in the basal metabolism of the body. A few studies have also used basal metabolism as an early predictor of obesity, especially when there is increased carbohydrate burning than intake.

Approximately 10 per cent of the energy of total energy transactions is utilised in the generation of heat and maintaining body temperature. This process is grossly under the control of the sympathetic nervous system and influenced by catecholamines. Thyroid hormones play the most important role in thermogenicity and hence this is one of the earliest treatments of obesity. The fat uncoupling proteins are another important factor to be considered in considering body thermoregulation. Several enzymes also play an important role in this.

2. *Physical activity:* Physical activity uses energy over basal metabolism. This happens at every movement of the body which spends energy. We know that weight and physical activity together determine the amount of energy spent. Expenditure of energy can be increased by increasing the physical activity of the body. In a typical scenario, the levels of physical activity (both exercise and routine) are difficult to be maintained by a person with growing ages. Of late, increased automatic labor has reduced the physical activity significantly at all levels. Hence, increasing and maintaining the energy expenditure level and accelerating the use of energy by exercise is most important.

All other reasons of obesity are linked to the same principle. Hormone effects, leptin disorders, thermodynamics, all act through the principle of retention and expense of fats. All these mechanisms work through the metabolic route.

Causes of Obesity

Causes of obesity can be divided under various headings:

A. Fundamental Life Credentials

1 Sedentary lifestyle, couch potatoes

2 Socio-economic status (too poor, too rich)

3 Lack of exercise

4 Female sex

5 Increasing age

B. Eating Habits

1. Over-eating
2. Junk food, canned food and drinks especially with acid controls and preservatives
3. Icy cold food and drinks
4. Alcoholic beverages
5. Excessive sugars, sweets, cola beverages
6. Excessive fats
7. Animal origin foods, condensed milk, refined foods

8. Irregular starvation followed by sudden eating

C. Hormonal or Endocrine Conditions

1. Diabetes
2. Hypothyroidism (myxedema)
3. Giagantism (growth hormone hyper-secretion)
4. Cushing's syndrome
5. Increased male estrogen / decreased testosterone
6. Dystrophic insulin
7. Pancreatic failure, pancreatitis
8. Growth hormone hyposecretion
9. Ovarian hormonal disorder (polycystic overian disease, etc)

D. Metabolic Causes

1. Leptin secretion disorder
2. Certain hypertrophying myopahties
3. Malnutrition
4. Post-surgical
5. Hyperlipidemia
6. Constipation

E. Genetic Causes

1. Family history
2. Down's syndrome
3. Cohen's syndrome
4. Laurence-Moon's or Bardet-Bield's syndrome

F. Psychological causes

1. Emotional disturbances, depression, increased self-esteem
2. Stress related complex
3. Anxiety neurosis related disorder
4. Obsessive compulsive disorder, bulimia

G. Kidney Disorders

1. Dropsy / anasarca / uric acid disorder
2. Renal failure
3. Nephritic syndrome (current or treated)

H. Miscellaneous

1. Rheumatism
2. Autoimmune conditions

I. Neoplastic

I. Lipomatosis

2. Cancer in early stages
3. Hyperplasia and hypertrophy of adipocytes
4. Insulinoma
5. Craniopharingioma

J. Iatrogenic

1. Post-pregnancy
2. Consumption of steroids for certain disease treatments
3. Consumption of oral contraceptives
4. Causes involving hypothalamus

K. Hepatic causes

1. Fatty liver in early stages
2. Gall stones

All these causes of obesity may or may not be interlinked with each other. Many causes work through a similar or related major mechanism. For example, all psychological causes but bulimia act through the mechanism of steroid and catecholamines secretion mechanism. Most of the hormones ultimately have an impact on the metabolism. There are certain uncommon causes and less specific causes which are mentioned along with these in Appendix II, at the end of this book.

Availability of energy more than required or use of energy less than available, apparently the same mechanism in two different directions, is a major cause for obesity. Effects of enzymes and hormones, malnutrition and hepatic causes contribute a major part to these causes. In developed countries, most of the obese people have malnutrition and related symptoms. Iron deficiency anemia, reduced bone density etc. are common accompanying syndromes.

Review and Recap

1. Regulation of fats and their metabolism in the body is done by fat storage or generation versus fat energy consumption. Approximately 25 percent of the total energy expenditure is at the basal metabolism level.

2. Thyroxin and exertion promote the utility of fat. This promoters fat storage of steroids (estrogen being the highest), somatostatin and catecholamines.

3. Obesity is caused if energy expenditure is less than energy consumption.

Chapter 3

Metabolic Causes of Obesity

Metabolic causes predominate the group of causes of obesity. Such metabolic causes of obesity include all direct fat metabolism related causes, most of the hormonal causes and food habit related causes. As discussed already, fat in the body is storage of energy. Various reasons for excessive storage are directly related to the mean energy consumption versus feeding. Catecholamines are responsible at the root level through their A and B type receptors for use or store of fats. Many enzymes, hormones and neuro-psychic factors regulate this process grossly. Eating more than required or malnutrition is a major metabolic cause. For this purpose let us understand first the metabolism of fat in the body.

Availability of Excessive Energy than Required:
First Law of Thermodynamics

As discussed under pathophysiology, this can be considered here in a specific mode to learn about the Evolution of obesity:

1. **Consuming more than required**

    i. *Eating more than the required quantity of food:*

    This may be a habit in many cases. Quantity and energy requirement in the food are the most ignored areas in almost every region of the world. Mostly, eating quality is very imbalanced and consumption of roughage is low. In this scenario, the food required to quench the appetite is also more than what is actually required for activity and hence over-eating by habit becomes a dominant cause of obesity.

    ii. *Eating energy rich food:*

    Eating energy rich foods, as discussed above is the most common and important cause of obesity. Eating rich foods such as cream in Europe, ghee in India, cheese in China, oils and coconut cream in coastal Asia and butter in almost all parts of the world, are common examples. Cereals very low in fiber and very high carbohydrates are also not uncommon. Eating cakes, chapaties, pastries and rice, which is majorly consumed by both vegetarians and non-vegetarians, itself is a strong source of excess energy. All junk foods are very rich in energy.

iii. *Eating disorders:*

Eating disorders such as bulimia and obsessive compulsive polyphagia make the patient eat more than what is required. This results in deposition of a lot of fat in the body.

iv. *Eating excess of sugars, sugar depositing materials:*

This point postulates a major disadvantage of globalisation and a few altered food habits. Food articles such as canned beverages, aerated drinks, etc. are rich in sugars. They are the major contributors to "insensible sugar intake" as we rarely care about the energy consumed from drinks. Furthermore, phosphoric acid, which is a major flavoring constituent of all cola drinks interferes with sugar metabolism thus leading to excessive sugar deposition and calcium depletion.

2. **Non-consumption of available energy**
   i. Lifestyle related non-consumption of the available energy is a major cause of central obesity in most of the sedentary lifestyle professionals. This is unfortunately a major reason for obesity in children where physical exercise is significantly reduced due to modified study and sports equilibrium pattern.
   ii. Low exercise or reduced profession related physical exertion indolent to exercise also results in obesity. Addiction to watching television is another cause in most developed and developing countries. Video game apparatuses have also gained lot of popularity as well. All these factors are thereby increasing the over all laziness factor. This significantly adds to the excessive fat deposition in a person's body. Although rhythmic and advanced exercise systems have developed and have been adopted, their use is yet not as wide as required.

3. **Material interfering with fat deposition metabolism**
   i. Icy cold food and drinks
   ii. Alcoholic beverages
   iii. Cola beverages
   iv. Animal origin foods and condensed milk

v. Canned foods and drinks especially those with acid controls and preservatives.

vi. Refined foods.

Unavailability of Enough Protein Energy

1. In developed countries, obesity is generally related to insufficient nutrition. This lack of nutrition is majorly due to a modification of the food habits — the food is low in fiber and protein material. Studies have demonstrated a direct correlation between protein levels in the body and fat metabolism. In case of lack of essential amino acids, fat deposition in the tissues increases.

2. In many developing regions, where food sources are low in proteins, obesity is related to protein energy malnutrition. It is especially seen in children having kwashiorkor – they have a classical central obesity with emaciation of the extremities.

Obesity Related to Fat Metabolism Influencing Factors

1. **Factors leading to lower fat consumption:**

   i. *Thyroid hormone deficiency:* Thyroid hormone deficiency due to any reason such as, primary or secondary hypothyroidism, low iodine intake, chlorosis or fluorsis, etc. leads to low fat consumption in the body. Thyroid hormone is a major cataboliser of body fat. In the absence or deficiency of this hormone, the basal metabolic rate falls. The fat mixed with a swelling-like condition due to thyroid hormone deficiency is called myxedema.

ii. *Irregular eating habits:* Irregular eating habits and frequent eating after a period of long fasting is one of the reasons which leads to lower consumption of fats.

iii. *Too vigorous and strong exercise:* When the exercise is very strong and fast, the brain, heart, kidneys and lungs have to work faster. Skin is over secreting. In this scenario, the body requires energy from a quicker source. This source cannot be fat because fat catabolism is a long procedure. Hence, in such cases, the body consumes its glycogen stores and the fat storage further increased.

2. **Diabetes:**

Diabetes and fat metabolism are multi-dimensionally related to each other. Its interference in fat metabolism constitutes a major morbidity in diabetic patients. Also, obesity and diabetes is very closely related to each other from many dimensions including this one.

3. Factors leading to excessive fat deposition

i. *Factors stimulating alpha adrenergic receptors in fat metabolism:*

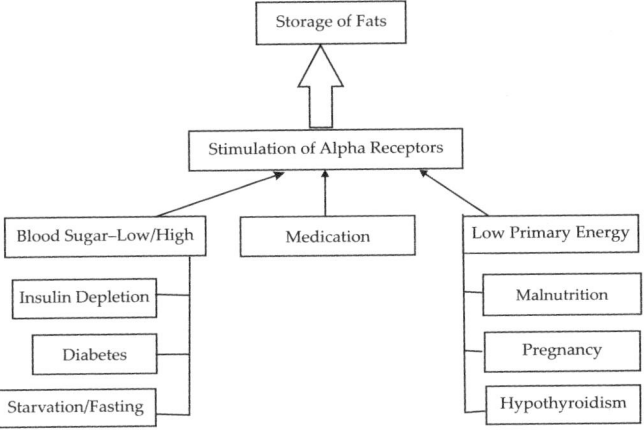

Fig, 3.1 Metabolic Causes of Fat Deposition

As discussed earlier, fat deposition in disorders or above mentioned factors are related to adrenalin stimulation. The two (alpha and beta) receptors stimulated by adrenalin have an exactly opposite actions on fat metabolism. Alpha receptor stimulation is related to fat deposition. The diagram above summarises the related metabolic causes.

ii. *Constipation:* Constipation causes reflexes to suppress intestinal mobility. This, in turn, pours a lot of amino acids into the lymphatics. Sluggish distended intestinal mass also leads to bulging of the abdominal belly, leading to central obesity.

iii. *Factors leading to muscles wasting:* This is a non-specific cause but has metabolic significance. Muscle wasting releases proteins from muscles which, in turn, causes increased amino acids leading to deposition of fatty acids in the body, mostly in the muscular and subcutaneous spaces.

iv. *Neoplastic:* Some tumours such as lipomas and cancers in the initial stages cause excessive deposition of fats. This is mainly due to secretion of some factors like tumour growth factors or tumour necrosis factor.

4. Leptin secretion disorder

Leptin is an indicator of fat stores in the body. Adipose tissue secretes leptin majorly, which is recognised by the brain and ultimately results in the modification of sensation of hunger or satiety and consumption of energy. The other sources of leptin include—placenta, ovaries, skeletal muscle, lower part of fundic gland of stomach, mammary epithelium, bone marrow, pituitary gland and liver.

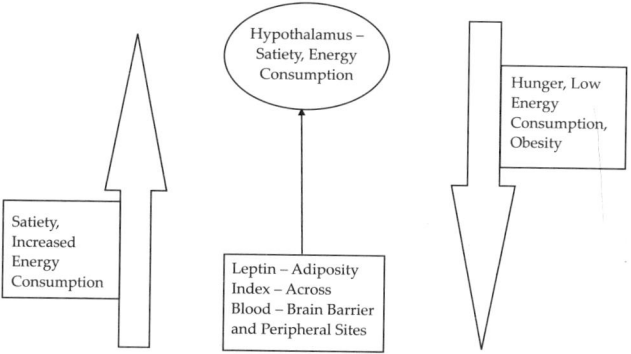

Fig 3.2 Role of Hormonal Controlers of Hunger and Satiety

Lower leptin levels in the body increase food intake and diminish energy consumption. This leads to obesity. Though leptin secreting disorder is related to genetic factors, there is not enough evidence of its solitary occurrence for making any confirmatory statement about its expression. There are many people with altered leptin levels without genetic changes. One more of the possibilities of leptin malfunctioning is functional leptin resistance. This mainly attributes to inability of leptin to cross blood brain barrier or inhibition of leptin related signals. The most common form of obesity has leptin levels below standard and is associated with hormonal dysfunction frequently.

Definitive treatment of leptin secreting disorder is supplement of leptin. Majorly due to insufficient data, anyhow, the treatment cannot be universalised. Hormonal treatment for the accompanying disorder is also an important part of the treatment. There are leptin supplements and leptin foods available for treatment of obesity. Considering leptin is a common factor of metabolic obesity, some commercials use letin as assured weight loss treatment (leptin is known as thinning hormone).

5. Certain hypertrophying myopathies

Hypertrophying myopathies include increase of weight and apparently involve myoskeletal leptin dysfunction and some of the parallel fatty acid regulation pathologies. There is a one to one correspondence in myopathy and obesity as both are causes and complications of each other. Fatty acid synthase is the enzyme that regulates formation of intrinsic fatty acids from other sources such as glucose. Excessive fatty acid synthase promotion leads to metabolic adipose tissue disorders in most cases and leads to obesity. An excess of gym, myotrophic exercises and consumption of artificial protein supplements are a few risk factors in this condition. There is no specific patho-physiology known and hence there is no definitive treatment for this condition.

Certain connective tissue disorders such as systemic lupus erythmatosus, autoimmune myosis or myopathy are responsible for this condition.

Among the probable treatments, moderating exercise especially gym and myotrophic exercises is very important. Leaving exercise suddenly or completely even gradually will lead to a myopathic situation where obesity may be one of the complications. Balancing the protein and fat intake is another very important aspect of the treatment. Sometimes, medical treatment that includes steroids or synthase antagonists, antihistaminics, etc. may be given, but no specific treatment has yet been jotted down.

6. **Post-surgical**

Post-surgical weight gain is mainly a lifestyle modification impact. There is modification in the lifestyle. Almost eighty women out of hundred in Asia and Africa, and almost thirty in proportion in Europe and America grow obese post child-birth. Higher metabolic state due to major repairs happening in the body and simultaneously low exercise levels are clearly two responsible factors.

Additionally, most communities have some or the other dietary customs for the post-surgical / post-delivery period. All these customary food articles have very high fat and myotrophying proteins.

Few Facts about Metabolic Obesity

a. Metabolic obesity is majorly either due to excessive energy supply or due to the non-consumption of the energy available.

b. Metabolic obesity is mainly central but may also be uniform.

c. Malnutrition may also lead to metabolic obesity.

d. More than half of the obese population has metabolic obesity.

e. Approximately only 10 per cent of the metabolically obese people are aware that they are obese.

f. Only about 5 per cent of the overweight population is aware about the various reasons and aids available to control increasing weight, without any underlying disease.

g. Only 3 per cent of the total population is aware of the hazards of metabolic obesity.

h. Obesity clinics are attended by only 15 per cent of the total projected attendance. Metabolic obesity attends there only in severe cases.

i. Most of us get signals from the body if we over eat. Some of us may experience hiccoughs when the stomach is full, immediately or after some time. Some may feel nausea, distention in the abdomen, hardness in the stomach region, food regurgitation, etc. Some may develop diarrhea or vomiting while the most of us ignore this.

The Balanced Diet

A balanced diet is the most important part of making one's life healthy. What you eat makes your personality, physical and even psychological to some extent. Let us first understand the major diet constituents, their sources and their function in the body. Also, we will need to understand where we spend the energy and how much extra energy do we store. Balancing one's diet and energy requirements is vital for managing one's health status.

The major contents of a balanced diet are:

1. **Carbohydrates:**

    i. Primary and quick source of energy (sugars). Glucose is primarily and mostly used by the muscles but it is the primary source of energy for the brain.

ii. Excess of carbohydrates are stored with a large quantity of water as glycogen in the skeletal muscles and the liver. Further excess of carbohydrates are stored as fats.

iii. Fructose is converted into glucose by the liver before it is used by the skeletal muscles, or it turns into triglycerides (it cannot be stored as glycogen).

2. Proteins:

i. These provide a source of basic materials for growth and repair, that is, development for all tissues of the body.

ii. They are used as a source of energy in some emergency cases.

iii. Most of the body's activities have proteins involved, in some way or the other. All the major secretions of the body such as— enzymes, hormones, immunity material and body's tissues, nerves, muscles or any type of cell, is made up of protein. Infact, we can say, anything and every thing in the body is protein.

iv. There are two major proteins—albumins and globulins, each having a defined role to play.

3. **Fats:**
   i. Provide a source of energy.
   ii. Contain fat soluble vitamins.
   iii. They can be stored in the body for a longer time in a larger volume.

4. **Vitamins:**

   These micro-nutrients are required for several health processes.

5. **Mineral salts:**

   These are required for various reasons in the body. Many minerals/salts may have a one to one correspondence with some tissue or organ, such as bones and teeth have a lot of calcium; blood (red blood corpuscles) contain iron.

6. **Fiber:**
   i. They make the indigestible bulk of food, and help the intestines function correctly.
   ii. Roughage is the main source of fibers which also contains some vitamins.

For being more specific, we have to understand more details of requirements of each of these nutrients in more details. Balanced diet is the one, which provides all the required energy and nutrients to the body.

Table 3.1 The Required Energy Nutrients of the Body

Nutrients	Daily Requirement	Source	Acceptable Macronutrient Distribution Range (AMDR)		
Carbohydrates	130 - 180 gm per meal	These all are names, this may not be a sentence construction. Only names are quoted. Sugars (free, row and in fruits, compounded as in drinks) Others (carbohydrates are commonly present in many components of food such as salads.)	45 – 65 per cent of the total meal quantity in a balanced Diet		
Proteins	30 – 50 gms per meal	Pulses, vegetables, fruits, milk, cheese, chassin, egg, soya bean and soya products	Children		Adults
			1-3 years	4-18 years	
			5-20	10-30	10-35
Fats		Oils, ghee, butter, cheese, animal fat, milk, oil seeds	Children		Adults
			1-3 years	4-18 years	
			30-40	25-35	20-35

(contd.)

(contd.)

Vitamins	There are several vitamins in the food; A, D, E and K are the fat soluble vitamins while C and B complex are water soluble vitamin.	The vitamin sources are described separately in the table below			
Minerals and Ions	The major minerals those are required for body's maintenance are calcium, iron, zinc an copper. Their intake in food must be taken carefully.	The mineral sources are described separately in the table below.			
Fibers	Quantity can be increased for supplement of restricted food.	Green leafy vegetables, roots, non-citrus fruits			25 – 35 per cent

(contd.)

(contd.)

| Water | 3 – 5 liters | Drinking water, liquids and some routine foods | | | |

Fat is a reservoir of energy. Hence, a low calorie diet will help to burn out the fat with even routine activity. Exercise, in addition, will help one to achieve the effect of weight loss faster. Principle of good diet management is to balance your diets on average summing up. For example, we take three diets in a day. Breakfast, Lunch and dinner. Some day, I am called for a dinner in a restaurant. I like Donuts, I eat three with a lot of cream on it. On top of that, there was also a round of special Indian desserts which has a lot of fat too. I was too full. Fine enough. I have now already stored the energy in the body that will suffice my 4 meals. But I cannot and should not starve myself. Hence I take a lot of green leafy vegetables, plain raw soups, fat free milk, fruits, fiber etc. I shall refrain from sweet beverages (cold or boiled) and another heavy food. This will continue till I reach the average energy intake of my meals including this heavy diet to my desired level. Approximately this will require my austere diets or six partially austere diets. Although we are calculative, we should not panic or be hypochondriac. Take it easy but not lightly.

Table 3.2 Vitamins, their Sources and Body's Vitamin Requirements

Vitamin	Physiological Action	Average Daily Requirement (Adults)	Deficiency Disease	Sources
Vitamin A	Eyes, skin	10,000 IU	Night blindness, xerophthalmia.	Cod liver oil, egg yolks, butter, raw whole milk, papaya, carrots, cashew nuts, muskmelon, mangoes.
Vitamin B1 (Thiamine)	Energy formation in cells, especially from carbohydrates.	10 – 50 mg	Weakness, fatigue.	Grapes, grapefruit, pork, sheath germ, pasta, peanuts, legumes, watermelon, oranges, brown rice, oatmeal, eggs, avocado, boysenberries, breadfruit, cheri-moya, dates, Guava, loganberries, mango, orange, pineapple, pomegranate, watermelon.

(contd.)

(contd.)

Vitamin B2 (Riboflavin)	Eyes, cell development, skin.	10 – 50 mg	Beriberi, eczema.	Milk, cottage cheese, avocados, tangerines, prunes, asparagus, broccoli, mushrooms, beef, salmon, turkey, banana, cherimoya, dates, grapes, lychee, mango, mulberries, passion fruit, pomegranate, prickly pear.
Vitamin B3 (Niacin)	Fat, protein and carbohydrate metabolism, nervous system.	25 mg	Nervousness, weakness.	Avocado, boysenberries, breadfruit, cherimoya, dates, guava, loganberries, lychee, mango, nectarine, passion fruit, peach, meats, poultry, fish, peanut butter, legumes, soybeans, whole grains, broccoli, asparagus, baked potatoes.

(contd.)

(contd.)

Vitamin B5 (Pantothenic Acid)	Energy, protein and carbohydrate metabolism.	25 - 150 mg		Avocado, black currants, breadfruit, cherimoya, dates, gooseberries, grapefruit, guava, pomegranate, raspberries, star fruit, watermelon, broccoli, brussel sprouts, butternut squash, corn, french beans, mushrooms, okra, parsnip, potatoes, pumpkin, spirulina spaghetti squash, squash – summer, squash - winter, sweet potato, fish, whole grain, mushrooms, peanuts, cashews, lentils, soybeans, eggs.
Vitamin B6	Brain, heart, immune system, protein metabolism.	50 – 200 mg		Fish, soybeans, avocados, lima beans, chicken, bananas, cauliflower, green peppers, potatoes, spinach, raisins.

(contd.)

(contd.)

Vitamin B9 (Folic Acid)	Heart, brain, red blood cell development.	400 – 800 mcg	Anemia, nervousness, weakness	Avocado, blackberries boysenberries, breadfruit, cherimoya, dates, guava, loganberries, lychee, mango orange, papaya, passion fruit pineapple, pomegranate, raspberries, strawberries, legumes, poultry, tuna, wheat germ, mushrooms, oranges, asparagus, broccoli, spinach, bananas, strawberries, cantaloupes.
Vitamin B12	Nerves, blood, tissue growth.	50 - 100 mcg		Salmon, eggs, cheese, swordfish, tuna, clams, mussels, oysters.
Biotin	Hair, skin, energy.	30 – 300 mcg		Peanut butter, eggs, oatmeal, wheat, gram, poultry, cauliflower, nuts, legumes.
Vitamin C	Immune system	250 – 2000 mg	Scurvy	Citrus fruit, strawberries, tomatoes, bell peppers, spinach, cabbage, melons, broccoli, kiwi fruit, raspberries.

(contd.)

(contd.)

Vitamin D	Bones, calcium absorption.	400 – 800 IU	Rickets, osteomalacia, Obesity	The major part of vitamin D is synthesised by skin in sunlight. Second major source is synthesised by kidney. Eggs, milk, butter, tuna and salmon are the external sources of vitamin D.
Vitamin E	Heart, immune system	200 – 400 IU	Obesity.	Oil, nuts, vegetable oils, wheat germ, mangoes, blackberries, apples, broccoli, peanuts, spinach, whole wheat.
Vitamin K	Blood clotting	20 – 60 mcg		Liver Synthesises Vitamin K in the body. Spinach, broccoli, brussel sprouts, cabbage, parsley, eggs, dairy products, carrots, avocados, tomatoes.
Mixed carotenoids	Immune system	5,000 – 15,000 IU		Carrots, pumpkin, sweet potatoes, spinach, butternut squash, tuna, cantaloupe, mangoes, apricots, broccoli, watermelon.

There are certain sources of vitamin having high energy content. Still, vitamins are extremely important for the maintenance of one's body. Hence, while designing a balanced diet, a lot of care should be taken that the energy, quantity, macronutrients and micronutrients are very well balanced. While making a diet for reducing obesity, it is especially important to include all vitamins in the required quantity in the dietary plan.

The other part of micronutrients is minerals and ions. These minerals and ions are important for the daily functioning of the body. Many of them play a vital role in physiological get going. The Table 3.3 below mentions various minerals, their roles, requirements and sources.

Table 3.3 Various minerals, their Roles, Requirements and Sources

Mineral	Physiological Sphere	Daily Requirement	Common Natural Sources
Calcium	Bones, teeth, muscle and nerve function, heart.	800 – 1,200 mg	Milk, cheese, yogurt, salmon, sardines with bones, broccoli, green beans, almonds, turnip greens, kale.
Magnesium	Blood pressure, nerve and muscle function, formation of enzymes.	400 – 600 mg	Molasses, nuts, spinach, wheat, germ, pumpkin seeds, seafood, dairy products, baked potatoes, broccoli, bananas.
Selenium	Immune system, prostate.	100 – 300 mcg	Meats, whole grain, dairy products, fish, shellfish, mushrooms, Brazil nuts.

(contd.)

(contd.)

Sodium	Fluid balance, nervous system function, kidneys.	2,400 mg	Salt, processed food, soy sauce (most people will not need to supplement their sodium intake, given the prevalence of sodium in our diets).
Potassium	Acid balance in body, fluid balance, hemodynamic, kidneys.	3,000 – 6,000 mg	Potatoes, avocados, bananas, yogurt, cantaloupe, spinach, mushrooms, milk, tomatoes.
Zinc	Immune system, prostate, wound healing, hair, gastrointestinal tract.	15 – 20 mg	Oysters, lean beef, wheat germ, seafood, lima beans, legumes, nuts, poultry, dairy products.
Phosphorus	Energy, bones, carbohydrate metabolism.	800 mg – 1,000 mg	Meats, fish, poultry, eggs, dairy products.
Manganese	Blood sugar, energy.	2 – 10 mg	Nuts, whole grains, legumes, tea, dried fruits, spinach, green leafy vegetables.
Molybdenum	Nitrogen metabolism, energy.	25 – 250 mcg	Legumes, meats, whole grains, milk, dairy products.
Chloride	Aids digestion, fluid balance.	750 mg	Foods with salt (most people will not have to supplement their chloride intake due to their high salt intake)

(contd.)

(contd.)

Chromium	Carbohydrate metabolism	50 – 200 mcg	Whole grains, broccoli, grapes, oranges, brown sugar, meats, black pepper, brewer's yeast, cheese.
Copper	Blood cells, connective tissue formation, liver and spleen	1.5 – 3 mg	Oysters, other shellfish, nuts, cherries, cocoa, mushrooms, gelatin, whole grains, eggs, fish, legumes.
Flouride	Tooth enamel	1.5 – 4 mg	Fluoridated water, fish, tea (most people do not have to supplement their fluoride intake due to fluoridation of the water supply).
Iodine	Proper thyroid function, basal metabolic rate.	150 mcg	Spinach, lobster, shrimp, oysters, milk, iodised salt.
Iron	Carries oxygen in blood, energy metabolism, formation and maturation of red blood cells.	10 – 20 mg	Clams, asparagus, meats, chicken, prunes, raisins, spinach, pumpkin seeds, soybeans, tofu.

Again, many mineral sources are associated with high energy content. When a balanced diet is being designed especially for weight loss, the commonest mistake is ignorance about the mineral intake. Hence, care should be taken for adequate intake of all essential minerals in all diets.

Do's of Metabolic Obesity

1. Take a balanced/modified balanced diet. A diet having all essential components of nutrition is very important for control of obesity. Very obese people need to reduce their weight and should have a programmed diet control. The weight loss diet is usually restricted on fats while it is rich in roughage and proteins.

2. Regularise exercise: Breathing and energy loss exercises should be gradually started and increased till the level of adequate calorie loss.

3. Evaluate the required energy intake and the actual intake, and modify the diet as required.

4. Visit a dietician especially if you are suffering from some metabolic syndrome.

5. Take a psychological counselling if you are suffering from obsessive disorder or bulimia.

6. Take enough amount of water.

Review and Recap

1. Metabolic obesity is caused when the energy intake is more than energy expenditure.

2. Leptin mechanism of satiety and hunger is responsible for stimulation of fat storage and fat consumption; catecholamines promote storage of fats in the body.

3. A balanced diet contains micronutrients such as vitamins and minerals and macronutrients such as carbohydrates, fats and proteins.

4. Fat is energy stored in the body. Excess of carbohydrates and fructose are stored as fats but fat cannot be used for glycogen synthesis, proteins are broken down for this purpose.

5. Adequate mineral and vitamin intake should be taken care of while designing a balanced diet, whether calories are restricted or regular.

6- Balancing the intake of energy with expenditure is very important for wise management of food intake, especially if some day the intake is more.

Chapter 4

Obesity and Underlying Disease

Underlying disease causes are very important to understand when we consider obesity and its management. There are some conditions which attribute to both causes and complications of obesity. The causes of obesity as described in chapter 2 have various classifications but grossly speaking, there are some curable underlying conditions and a few are non-curable. Conditions pertaining to genetic reasons are non-curable. Certain other systems, especially endocrine system has a direct impact on obesity and metabolism, which needs to be treated medically, to manage the obesity related to these conditions.

Endocrine System and Obesity

The endocrine system and the hormones have a direct effect on fats consumption, deposition and restriction. The endocrine system consists of:

1. Pituitary (anterior and posterior)
2. Thyroid
3. Thymus
4. Pancreas
5. Adrenal (cortex medulla)
6. Gonads (males – testes; females – ovaries)

Hypothalamus controls the secretary function of all hormones via the Hypothalamus-Pituitary axis.

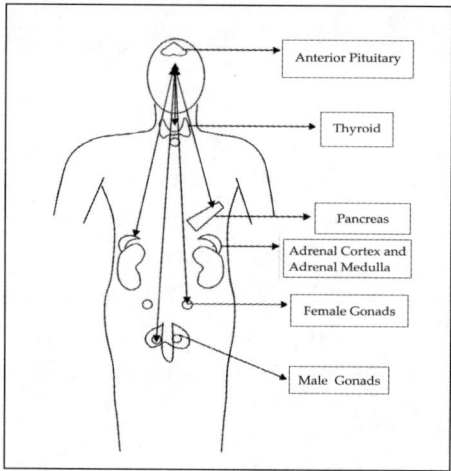

Fig. 4.1 Hypothalamus Control of the Secretary Function

The following Table 4.1 summarises hormones of various endocrine glands and their effect on the metabolism of fats. Once we understand the role of various hormones in fat metabolism, we start considering various diseases which may cause obesity from these hormonal causes. This information is vitally important in all cases dealing with obesity, for yourself or for others, for unless the hormones are balanced, weight management would not be possible.

Table 4.1 Hormones of Various Endocrine Glands and Their Effect on the Metabolism of Fats

Gland	Hormones having Impact on Fat Metabolism / Deposition	Effect on Fat Metabolism
Pituitary – Anterior	Growth hormone (GH)	Growth hormone promotes lipolysis. While doing so, it promotes stability of muscle proteins.
		Growth hormone or Somatotropin maintains glucose within normal ranges.
	Adreno-corticotropic hormone (ACTH)	ACTH is responsible for secretion of corticosteroids, the hormones of suprarenal gland.
	Thyroid stimulating hormone (TSH)	TSH stimulates thyroid hormone secretion, which increases fat consumption.

(Contd.)

(contd.)

Pituitary–Posterior	Vasopressin	Vasopressin, also called anti diuretic hormone, can rarely impact fat metabolism, mainly through its action on water and electrolytes in the body.
Thyroid	Thyroxin (T4) Tri-iodothyronine (T3) – this works as T4 only	Thyroid hormones lead to mass breakdown of fat, its mobilisation and increased fatty acid concentration in plasma. It also leads to consumption of fat and its use for energy. Increasing carbohydrate breakage also occurs simultaneously under the influence of thyroid hormones and thus it increases the basal metabolic rate.

(contd.)

(contd.)

Pancreas	Insulin	Insulin causes conversion of excess glucose into fat and promotes storage in the cells. Insulin promotes synthesis of fatty acids in the liver. Insulin inhibits breakdown of fat in adipose tissue, it has a fat sparing effect.
	Glucagon	Promotes breakdown of fat and gluconeogenesis. Increasing blood glucose levels is the main role of glucagon.
Suprarenal Glands (Cortex)	Glucocorticoids	They cause stimulation of gluconeogenesis in the liver which leads to inhibition of glucose uptake in muscle and adipose tissues. This causes fatty acid mobilisation in the tissues. By stimulation of fat breakdown in adipose tissues and restriction of glycogen entry into adipose tissues, it increases blood glucose levels.

(contd.)

(contd.)

Suprarenal Glands–Medulla	Adrenalin and noradrenalin	Adrenalin and noradrenalin both stimulate lipolysis in fat cells, but also respond to hypoglycemia and can lead to fat storage.
Gonads	Estrogen	Causes fat deposition, especially in female sexual area.
	Testosterone	Causes fat deposition in male sexual areas, but not in general.

With this background of physiology, let us consider the common hormonal causes of obesity:

1. Diabetes
2. Hypothyroidism (mexedema)
3. Gigantism (growth hormone hypersecretion)
4. Cushing's syndrome
5. Increased male estrogen
6. Dystrophic insulin disorder
7. Pancreatic failure or pancreatitis
8. Ovarian hormonal disorder (polycystic ovarian disease, etc.)

Diabetes

Diabetes has a multifaceted relation in both directions with obesity. It is a cause as well as a complication. Here, we will discuss diabetes as a cause of obesity. Diabetic people face a lot of blood sugar level imbalances. This is a primary factor for the stimulation of fat burning and reduction of weight in the initial phase. This may be from insulin resistance initially. In the later phases, diabetes leads to stimulation of alpha adrenergic receptors resulting in diminution of insulin activity diminution. Both these conditions tend to increase fat deposition. There are various reasons for metabolic disturbances in diabetes. A few diabetics may face hypoglycemia or ketosis; both these conditions will lead to further obesity.

The second aspect of relationship of diabetes and obesity is that obese patients commonly exhibit insulin resistance and glucose intolerance. The normal insulin regulation pathway of direct glucose uptake is hence diminished. The glycogen storage is diminished in quantity. However, other insulin-mediated pathways like hepatic conversion of glucose to triglycerides still persist. This leads to glucose ingestion in obesity for increased fat stores, and a vicious cycle is initiated. Insulin resistance and its consequences are reversible with reduced fat stores. New theories of reducing carbohydrate intake to achieve weight reduction are based upon this fact.

Oral hypoglycemic agents used for the treatment of diabetes have a low impact on fat deposition. These agents allow reduction of blood sugar and hence some times alternative insulin fat conversion mechanisms may be activated by them. These oral hypoglycemic agents have a little tendency of stimulation of alpha receptors. Hence they may trigger activation of triglycerides formation or hyperplasia of the adipose tissue.

A very carefully balanced diet is a vital part of diabetes related obesity treatment. Understanding diet and medicine needs, blood sugar levels and appetite satisfying quantity is important.

Do's of Diabetes and Related Obesity

1. Test your blood sugar regularly.
2. Follow up with your physician and dietitian regularly.
3. Manage your food according to your work and exercise, and medicinal dose.
4. Monitor your weight and lipid periodically.
5. Add exercise to your routine.

Hypothyroidism

Thyroid Hormones and Fat Consumption

Thyroid hormones are responsible for fat metabolism in the body majorly. The thyroid hormone called Thyroxin, also known commonly as T4 hormone has a direct impact on fat consumption in the body. It is, therefore, important to understand the functions of thyroid hormones before proceeding further to the diseases of the thyroid gland.

Function of Thyroid Hormones

1. Act on nearly every cell in the body, helps proper development and differentiation of all human cells.

2. Regulates protein, fat and carbohydrate metabolism by human cells; increases fat consumption and affects protein synthesis.

3. Along with growth hormone, helps regulate long bone growth and nerve cell maturation.

4. Increases the body's sensitivity to catecholamines.

5. Stimulates vitamin metabolism.

6. Numerous physiological and pathological stimuli influence thyroid hormone synthesis.

7. Thyroid hormones lead to heat generation in humans.

8. Thyroid hormones increase the basal metabolic rate by stimulating diverse metabolic activities in most tissues.

   a. *Lipid Metabolism:* Thyroid hormones stimulate fat mobilisation, subsequently increasing plasma fatty acids concentrations. They also accelerate oxidation of fatty acids in many tissues. They reduce plasma concentrations of cholesterol and triglycerides.

   b. *Carbohydrate Metabolism:* Thyroid hormones stimulate all the aspects of carbohydrate metabolism. It enhances the insulin-dependent entry of glucose into cells. Increased gluconeogenesis and glycogenolysis to generate free glucose are also stimulated by thyroid hormones.

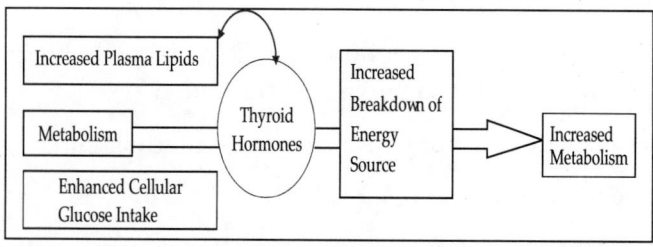

Fig. 4.2 Carbohydrate Metabolism

Thyroid hormone secretion is based upon feedback mechanism, for which a regulatory stimulus via the pituitary is generated in the form of increased or decreased TSH secretion.

As thyroid hormones promote consumption of fats, mainly, lower thyroid hormone levels cause obesity.

Table 4.2 Conditions of Low Thyroid Hormone Secretion

Type	Description
Primary- Thyroid Causes	1. Hashimoto's thyroiditis (an autoimmune disease). 2. Radioiodine therapy for hyperthyroidism. 3. Lithium-based mood stabilisers. 4. Insufficient iodine intake.
Secondary-Pituitary	1. Suppression of thyroid stimulating hormone (TSH) secretion. 2. Damage to the pituitary gland, as by a tumour, radiation or surgery.
Tertiary-Hypothalamus	Insufficient thyrotropin-releasing hormone (TRH) secretion.

Obesity Related to Thyroid

Obesity related to hypothyroidism is due to non-consumption of fat. Myxedema, the term for weight gain from thyroid hormone deficiency indicates deposition of fat, retention of water and muscle relaxation.

There are other associated key diagnostic symptoms or associated symptoms of thyroid related obesity:

1. Poor muscle tone
2. Fatigue
3. Increased sensitivity to cold
4. Depression, loss of memory
5. Muscle cramps and joint pain
6. Thin, brittle finger nails and hair
7. Paleness
8. Decreased sweating; dry, itchy skin
9. Weight gain and water retention, swelling all over the body
10. Decreased heart rate.
11. Constipation

Treatment of Hypothyroidism

1. Replenishment of thyroid hormones:

    i. Thyroid hormones (T3 + T4 or alone T4) from animal origin – desiccated

    ii. Use of the synthetic analogue of thyroxin (T4)

2. Increasing Iodine intake to adequate levels

Do's of Thyroid Disease

1. Have a regular follow up and check up of unbound T4.
2. Maintain your weight and diet.
3. Maintain your iodised salt intake at an adequate quantity.
4. Take your medication regularly.
5. Do not overexert.

Facts about Thyroid Related Obesity

1. Thyroid related obesity is not a fatness but is a disease – swelling.
2. Thyroid related obesity, cold intolerance and low heart rate can be fatal.

Cushing's Syndrome – Hypersteroidism

Cushing's syndrome is increased levels of cortisol steroid hormone in the blood.

Cushing's syndrome can be of two types – exogenous and endogenous, depending upon the source of increased steroid hormone. If steroids are from outside it is exogenous; which is more common; and if from within the body, it is called endogenous.

Causes

Exogenous

1. Medical prescription of glucocorticoids prescribed for treatment of asthma, rheumatoid arthritis or as an immunosuppressant after an organ transplant is very common.

2. Hormonal contraceptives in inadequately high doses.

3. Administration of synthetic ACTH is less common.

Endogenous

1. *Derangement of cortisol secretion system:*

   i. *Pituitary:* Pituitary ACTH stimulates the release of cortisol from the adrenal glands. Some pituitary conditions lead to increased ACTH production which in turn leads to increased cortisol production. For example, benign pituitary adenoma.

ii. *Adrenal:*
    a. Adrenal gland tumours.
    b. Hyperplastic adrenal glands.
    c. Adrenal glands with nodular adrenal hyperplasia.
iii. *Ectopic ACTH Production:* ACTH produced out of pituitary-adrenal system that affects the adrenal glands such as in (paraneoplastic) small cell lung cancer.

Physiology of Secretion of Cortisol

Corticotropin-releasing hormone (CRH) is released from the paraventricular nucleus (PVN) of the hypothalamus, which stimulates the pituitary gland to release adreno-corticotropin (ACTH). ACTH stimulates the adrenal cortex for the release of cortisol. This mechanism works upon feedback system. In case there is a tumour in the pituitary or adrenal cortex, or excessive intake of steroids, this mechanism is disturbed leading to Cushing's syndrome.

Steroids and Fat Metabolism

All steroids including gonad hormones have a very specific action on fats.

Signs and Symptoms

1. Rapid weight gain, particularly central obesity – the trunk and face with sparing of the limbs.

2. Lipodystrophy – formation of fat pads along the collar bone and on the nape of the neck (buffalo hump).

3. Moon face, that is, round face.

4. Acne, especially on the face.

5. Excess sweating.

6. Telangiectasia (dilation of capillaries).

7. Thinning of the skin, mucus membranes, leading to bruises, dryness.

8. Dark, black, purple or red striae, a result of stretch marks of thin, dry and weakened skin, followed by subsequent hemorrhage.

9. Hirsutism – male pattern, facial hair growth.

10. Other endocrine systems are affected like, insomnia, reduced libido, impotence, amenorrhea and infertility, psychological disturbances, depression and anxiety.

11. Hypertension – increased blood pressure.

12. Hyperglycemia – increased blood sugar level.

Treatment

1. Careful tapering off and eventually stopping steroids if consuming them (therapeutic or anabolic as a dope).

2. Adrenal adenoma, ACTH-secreting pituitary adenoma to be removed.

3. Removal of adrenals to eliminate production of excess cortisol may be one of the choices in severe cases.

Obesity Related to Steroids

Cortical related obesity is mainly central where as estrogen related obesity is in buttocks, breasts and belly. Testosterone does not have much of a direct effect on deposition of fats. In fact, low testosterone may lead to obesity. Polycystic ovarian disorder is also one of the common conditions where obesity is present; it may be associated with estrogen secretion modifications. Cortisol analogues are most commonly found causes of obesity.

Facts about Steroid Related Obesity

1. Most common cause of steroid related obesity is misuse of steroids for various reasons, especially by athletes and body builders.

2. Steroids are the most misused drugs in the Indian subcontinent.

3. Steroid related obesity is commonly due to the external use of steroids than internal diseases.

Hormonal Causes: Review and Recap

1. Major hormonal causes of obesity are: Hypothyroidism, Cushing's syndrome and diabetes. Minor causes include pituitary imbalance.

2. All hormonal disturbances that lead to obesity, essentially work through the metabolic pathway but cannot be treated by diet alone. Careful treatment and dietary regulation is required.

3. Many hormonal diseases of adulthood are not fully curable, but the related obesity can be controlled very well.

Genetic Disorders and Obesity

Genetic causes include hereditary and chromosomal causes. All these causes, other than non-chromosomal familial obesity are incurable. In all these cases we have to satisfy ourselves by palliation alone, and reduce the weight carefully. In many conditions, there are other very serious conditions associated with the disorder. All we can do here is improve the quality of life and reduce the impact of obesity in the whole syndrome. These causes are:

1. Family history
2. Down's syndrome
3. Cohen's syndrome
4. Bardet Biedl syndrome

1. Family History

Familial obesity is a common condition. Familial obesity in common language may also be taken as hereditary obesity. This pertains to the traits running across generations. Some hereditary traits that people carry include rheumatic diathesis, lithiatic diathesis, phlegmatic diathesis, these people tend to be obese in many cases. All this is the familial contribution to one's built.

Pathogenesis of Familial Obesity

Single neucleopeptide polymorphism is a common cause of familial obesity. This may be expressed since birth, at puberty or adolescence. Prohormone convertase disorder, an enzyme that helps expression of proper chromosomal information, is one of the commonly suspected pathology for transmission of obesity from one generation to the other. Prohormone convertase is an enzyme that helps expression of proper chromosomal information. There are certain predispositions such as hypothyroidism in the family history or a preload of diabetic, commonly showing the tendency to grow obese.

Treatment

Familial obesity, if not due to a specific disorder, can be controlled with proper diet, exercise and careful weight management. Training for diet/exercise control is necessary for familial obesity tendency carrying individuals. If the individuals are carrying a diathesis prone to obesity, respective care for such causes and if required their treatment will be required.

The discussion on diet and exercise is more extensive in the following chapter. Treatment of predispositions needs to be constitutional. In modification of diet, all food that exaggerates the predisposition including diathesis should be avoided. There are certain spices helping to resolve the rheumatic, diabetic, etc. predispositions. These spices should be included in the food. There are some medicines in the herbal and homeopathic systems of medicine which take care of these predispositions. If the predispositions are more severe and expressive in acute exacerbations, proper treatment of these predispositions should cure the tendency for obesity also. However, diet and exercise is inevitable in all cases.

Other genetic disorders are almost non-curable conditions as there is some major genetic pattern variation. These three genetic disorders are mainly developmental or birth defects and along with obesity, have various other systemic defects.

2. Cohen's Syndrome

Cohen's syndrome is an uncommon condition; caused by mutations in the VPS13B gene (commonly called the COH1 gene). It is inherited in an autosomal recessive pattern, having both genes in each cell have mutations.

Signs and Symptoms

1. Developmental delay
2. Mental retardation
3. Microcephaly (small head size)
4. Hypotonia (weak muscle tone)
5. Progressive myopia (short sightedness)

6. Retinal dystrophy (degeneration of the light-sensitive tissue in the retina)

7. Hypermobility (unusually large range of movement) of joints

8. Thick hair and eyebrows

9. Long eyelashes

10. Unusually shaped, down-slanting and wave-shaped eyes

11. Nasal tip bulbous

12. Between the nose and the upper lip, there is a smooth or shortened area

13. Prominent upper central teeth

14. Open-mouth appearance

15. Neutropenia (low levels of white blood cells of a particular type)

16. Extremely friendly behaviour

17. Obesity that develops in late childhood or adolescence. Typically around the abdomen, sparing arms and legs, hands, feet and fingers

Treatment

No specific or curative treatment. Early diagnosis and management is the key.

For management of obesity, a proper diet is very important. Balanced diet with low calories is going to be the key. There are very high chances of muscle wasting in this condition as there are several associated conditions which may do so. The diet planned for these individuals should, hence be protein rich.

Tummy tuition may be very important as the obesity is mainly around the abdomen, usually sparing the limbs.

3. Bardet-Biedl Syndrome

BBS is a pleiotropic disorder (one gene change influences many changes in the series) having variable expressions with a wide range of clinical presentations.

Conventionally, there are twelve genes responsible for the disease. These genes, when mutated and cloned, lead to BBS. The BBS proteins are gene products encoded by these BBS genes. If it sounds too technical, it can be simplified as the basal body and the hairlike structures on them called cilia have these proteins in a particularly "encoded" form. This coded information will lead to expression of the BBS and disorder in cilia and basal body. Such proteins are also found in intraflagellar transport (IFT), which is a two way protin transportation within cilia. As a result of this abnormal protein present in cilia, wide range of symptoms develop in BBS patients. Abnormalities of cilia are known to produce a wide range of symptoms including those commonly seen in BBS patients.

Symptoms / Features

1. Visual loss preceded by night blindness since childhood.
2. Polydactyly (more number of digits – fingers and toes).
3. Obesity of trunk from infancy.
4. Learning difficulties.
5. Male hypogenitalism and female genitourinary malformations.
6. Renal dysfunctions (main cause of disease and deaths).

There is a very wide range of symptoms in this syndrome. No specific treatment is available.

Even management of obesity is very difficult in this case due to psychological problems and many associated critical conditions. Also, the age is comparatively very young to manage the obesity. In this case, all that one can do is help the person consume as healthy a diet as he can.

Genetic Obesity: Review and Recap

1. All genetic causes are irreversible conditions and have linked obesity that is very hard to manage and reduce.

2. Familial obesity is manageable to an extent with diet and exercise control besides great efforts and determination.

3. There are added disadvantages of genetic factors and other symptoms in this group of obesity causes.

Psychological Causes

Psychology Behind Hunger and Eating

The psychology of hunger and eating starts with a motivation to eat. This part is significantly complex. The primary part of hunger – motivation, is its biological aspect. The internal mechanism of the body regulates finely the quantity and quality of food required. Hunger is not just a matter of an empty stomach , but a desire to eat a variety of foods of different tastes is out of some additional needs and has psychological aspect to it. Hypothalamus is the basic organ of the body, especially the ventromedial nucleus, which restricts food intake, while the lateral hypothalamus stimulates. Usually it works through a 'weight set mechanism', optimising itself to a weight level of the body. Depending upon various hormones and metabolic activity, this weight set stimulates appetite via the hypothalamus.

Cultural and Social Impact

The intellect of man is one factor making him social and inducing social customs in him. In addition to the biological factors of hunger, the mechanism of eating motivation is highly impacted by the social and cultural customs. For example, sweets are an inevitable part of India and Asia. Irrelevant of exercise levels, the quantum of food intake is usually the same. Thus, here we all are custom impacting the hunger psychology. Grooming, has some or the other impact on our food, which is also an important contribution towards hunger psychology resulting in some particular desires and aversions. Thus, the foods which are hogged and while foods we do not like are rejected, irrelevant of their nutritional value.

Roots of Obesity

The psychological roots of obesity have various radicals. One theory of weight gain suggests that many human beings suppress natural hunger and satiety impulse due to socio-psychological and customary eating impulses. For example, even after having a full meal to the front of a belch, most of us cannot resist if some tempting filler or dessert or some favourite delicacy is offered. More so, people who intend to be indolent in doing any work for eating (such as shelling the nuts in experiment of Neisbett 1968), are tending to grow obese faster. All junk food eaters are commonly obese – the explanation is by this theory.

Some other wing of opinions advocates shifting of the weight set point with adaptation of the current weight by the body. For example, an initially lean person starts eating more and gains weight. Gradually, this new weight to which he has become comfortable is set to be a new reference point for the body and 'weight set mechanism' for hunger and satiety stimulation is reset to the food need for this point. Sometimes this weight set point gets stuck at high, which maintains the obesity. Eventually this may lead to obsession or tendency of a person to keep insulting natural satiety impulse of the body. Thus the obesity is aggravated in them.

In fact the first theory (socio-psychological) and second (bio-psychological) are true in most conditions in the same individual, whereas rarely only one applies, or both fail. But practically, the social and behavioural aspect of eating notion contributes a lot of value to obesity.

The 'Weight set mechanism'

Weight set mechanism is one of the most important aspect to knows but it has a limited practical applicability. This mechanism is stated by some experience driven principles and involves physiological explanation.

If observed, person's weight unless interfered with imbalances, is relatively stable. This pertains to the person's physiology by achieving a balance between gain and expenditure of energy, as discussed before. This physiology considers a particular state of weight and adiposity as a standard. All the actions of the body are then set about maintaining this weight as a standard point. If a person eats less, instead of releasing the energy from adipose tissue, it gives signals of hunger. And if one overeats for a day, he will not be hungry at the next meal despite being thin. This physiological standardisation of the weight by one's weight is called 'weight set' which, more or less, is a psychological mechanism.

Resetting 'weight set point' is possible and this is usually the aim of a person's ideal diet plan. The planned diet should have a stomach filling quantity with less energy. Due to the weight set, initially this weight set will lead to an increased desire to eat. Where, again some protein and carbohydrate containing food should be taken. Gradually, release and consumption of fat will start and the weight will reduce. After achieving the target weight, the quantity of food should start reducing very slowly and the new 'weight set point' will be set in on the new reduced weight. Very careful and determinative action from the dietician and patient both, are required to deploy a weight set mechanism for effective weight loss tool.

Psychological Causes of Obesity

The psychological causes of obesity are divisible into four major groups:

1. Emotional: Emotional disturbances, increased self esteem.

2. Stress and stress related complex.

3. Anxiety neurosis, depression and related disorders.

4. Obsessive compulsive disorder, bulimia.

All four groups are interlinked to each other in most of the cases. Many times these remain unnoticed as non-sensible causes. The obesity so caused becomes an additional factor for aggravation of any such disorder. Some causes are working directly on hyper-nutrition for example, bulimia.

Bulimia

This is an eating disorder where the affected person eats incredibly large amount of food. Following this, there is generally a feeling of guilt or depression. The person also tends to induce vomiting or consume purgatives. Although it is not necessary for a bulimia case to be obese, this is not uncommon.

Bulimia may be due to various reasons but one of its important a symptoms is bulimia nervosa which is of purging type or non-purging type.

Signs and Symptoms

1. Recurrent, episode-wise binge eating.
2. Feeling that he cannot control eating in an episode.
3. Eating a larger amount.
4. Eating in discreet periods.

5. Reflex compensatory behaviour (usually to induce weight loss).

6. It is more common in males and late adolescents or young adults.

In purging type of bulimia nervosa, there may be self induced vomiting, misuse of drugs such as laxatives, diuretics, hormones, etc.

Causes

1. Exact cause is not yet clear.
2. Neurotrasmitter system abnormalities in pituitary, gland and hypothalamus.
3. Socio-psychological and cultural desires about being fit.
4. Obesity, infact, is one of the major causes of bulimia nervosa.
5. Psychological preoccupation about the weight.
6. Family history.

Complications

1. Dehydration, malnutrition, electrolyte unbalance disorder.
2. Sudden episodes of increase or decrease in weight.

3. Depression and melancholy.
4. Suppressed or low flow menses.
5. Cardiac arrhythmia.
6. Sometimes persistent swelling on distal body parts.

Emotional Factor and Obesity

As discussed before, emotions have an impact on the hunger of a person. Appetite also has its linked emotions related to environment and company. Liking and disliking food in general or some particular item is also a set of emotions.

Emotional Disturbances and Hunger Increase

Almost every fifth person's hunger is stimulated by peaks of emotion such as—nervousness, anxiety, depression, cheer, enthusiasm, aphrodisium, fright (not fear, as fright has no insecurity linked with it; for example, mood while watching a horror movie), insecure feeling, melancholy, dissatisfaction, etc. Anxiety, depression and obsession are discussed separately for their larger spectrum and specific mechanism. All other emotions are considered for all practical purposes under emotional bundle. Hoggin on one type of food that is liked and rejecting other type of food that is disliked is also an emotional constituent of food psychology. This factor has an important role to play in causing obesity. For a particular type of food or taste is also an emotional factor of obesity. Some people will never eat bitter gourd or a bottle gourd despite knowing its nutritional value or its contribution to health; this reflects its best example.

Self Esteem and Hunger

Self-esteem and obesity correlation has gained significantly high attention from many psychologists for several reasons. Theoretically, self esteem and obesity has a cycle. Lower self-esteem can lead a stigma for obesity, probably due to discrimination. Considering a fact that leanness is attractive, discrimination of obese people (Primary obesity) and obesity in discriminated people (Secondary obesity) are cause complement to each other. Higher self-esteem may not be enough to keep away from obesity though. The problem with self esteem and perversion of hunger complex has commonly increased, especially in American children.

Anxiety, Stress and Related Complex

Stress is commonly blamed for weight loss in a person. Vice versa, stress increasing weight of a person, with or without increasing the appetite. This works in two ways, first the psychological aspect – the emotional factor increases hunger. The second way is hormonal. Stress is known to increase steroids especially cortisol in the body. This increased cortisol level if continued for a long enough time is sufficient to induce obesity. Obesity is more common in stress related complex where severe hormonal disturbances and metabolic influences of such stress are moderate to severe. This may initially even cause loss of weight but in the long term will cause weight gain.

Depression

Depression has no specific definition per se, when it comes to expression of the diseases. Simple disappointed mood to severe disturbances in physiology of perception as in cases of psychosis is an extensive extent of the depression. Clinically speaking, depression cannot be defined beyond a set of symptoms, where extreme sad mood with or without irritability is characteristically present.

Causes and features of depression are various. There are several primary and secondary reasons for weight gain in depressive disorders. Depression, physiologically involves a chemical imbalance in the brain, may be due to the stimulation of the depression nucleus. This may also effect the hypothalamus and leptin secretion. Tendency to eat, habitual alcoholism, consuming large doses of caffeine, ingesting heavy food frequently and repeated partying to boost the mood, leads to obesity. A reasonably good frequency is found, amongst the depression patients for abnormal cravings, more or less maniacal.

Also, sometimes there is treatment related obesity, such as in cases where the patient is told to consume food of his liking. Some lithium effective antidepressant drugs, also tend to make the patient obese. Nevertheless, there is no scope for discontinuance of the treatment, hence obesity in such patients cannot be controlled.

Obsessive Compulsive Disorders

Obsession is a habit of unreasonably performing (or even repeating) some act and when it is added with psychologically induced compulsion, it takes the form of obsessive compulsive disorder. Obsessive compulsive disorders have several heads as has been already discussed. There are a few obsessions which rule most of us in some way or the other. Taking three meals a day conventionally, whether hungry or not, is a type of faint obsession. Use of fats on some foods such as soup is more of obsession than logic.

A few obsessions are far beyond just being obsessions and take the shape of disorder, especially if the act is repeated and is superimposed with compulsive psychology. Eating obsessive compulsive disorders are faintly different than an eating disorder. Many times, the difference is in the cause. Another disorder is the guilty feeling of bulimia, due to which usually emenogauges or laxatives are misused.

Treatment of Psychological Causes of Obesity

Usually the psychological causes of obesity are too rare to present to an obesity or psychiatry clinic. Many such patients are convinced of being normal and feel no need of treatment for themselves. Whenever such a case is detected, the first aim is counselling.

Line of Treatment

1. Counselling:

i. By a clinical psychologist.

ii. By a dietician.

2. Medical treatment for underlying condition by a psychiatrist.

3. Reconfirmations about presence or absence of various associated diseases, and if present their treatment.

Psychology and Weight Loss

Dr Robert Feldman, in his unique work 'Understanding Psychology' has meticulously compiled guidelines for psychological aspects of weight loss. The crux of the writing is listed below:

1. **Determination:**
   i. Understand that there is no easy way to lose weight.
   ii. Permanent changes are required to lose and maintain lost weight.
   iii. Life time commitment to eat less and changing eating habits is required.
   iv. Strict balance in quantity and nutrient quality of food to be achieved.

2. **Setting reasonable goals:**
   i. A preset goal is required.
   ii. Do not try to lose too much weight quickly.

3. **Exercise:**
   i. Weight set point theory suggests – it may set your optimum weight to low, will decrease your general requirement.

ii. Exercise helps burning fat, as well as set less appetite.

iii. Will help feel good (especially in depressed subjects – due to endorphins).

4. **Decrease influence of external social stimuli on eating behaviour:**

i. Serve a smaller portion of food for yourself.

ii. Leave table instead of waiting for dessert.

iii. Restrict eating snacks (even peanuts, potato chips, etc.). Do not even buy and store them.

iv. Keep tempting food hidden, wrapped in opaque foils so that you cannot see them.

5. **Avoid fad diet:**

    Do not go by fad and fashion about food, including liquids.

6. **Do not feel guilty if you fail to lose weight:**

    i. Inability to lose weight may not be a failure in life.

    ii. Given obesity pattern may have different reasons.

7. **If in a paradox, avoid dieting in the first place:**

i. Help yourself manage averages of diet related energy.

ii. Prefer being slow and steady.

Psychology and Obesity: Review and Recap

1. Psychological factors explain obesity with 'weight set theory' and related physiology. The weight set point can be reset by systematic efforts and integral work up in the same line.

2. There are certain psychological factors responsible for over eating or hormonal imbalances and subsequently obesity. These factors are related to self esteem, anxiety, depression and eating disorders.

3. Psychological counselling helps inevitably in weight loss and weight management, in particular–determination.

4. It is important to have determination; set measurable targets and control at the point of start itself, such as controlling the purchase of snacks.

5. Psychology of obesity is usually related to social depression and added obesity driven from it adds more.

Renal, Neoplastic, Hepatic and Cardiac Causes of Weight Gain

The reason for writing weight-gain instead of obesity is swelling. Swelling is one of the most important reasons of weight-gain, which is more commonly confused with obesity, in all these three conditions. In fact, there are no reasons of obesity among heart disease, rare causes in kidney and only a few conditions relating to the liver.

Early stages of fatty liver or hepatic cirrhosis lead to increased weight. This may be due to either the death of some fat cells impacting body's fat index or due to loss of a proper fat metabolism. There are some chemical mediators in processes such as tumour necrosis factor, released in fatty liver and in neoplasm (discussed under causes of obesity), which seems to be the prima facie responsible for interference in the signals of body's adequate weight and hunger satiety. Cancers in early stages like lipomas, are examples of these.

In many patients of cholecystitis (inflammation of the gall bladder) and gall stones, obesity is observed. This problem is but a 'hen first or egg first' puzzle in most cases, where simultaneously both ailments are reported to a clinic. Obesity and excessive fat metabolism is a cause as well as a complication of gall stones. Same is true in converse.

Post-nephritic edema is commonly observed but this needs medical management of instead considering it just obesity. The reason behind such obesity may be as serious as progressive renal failure in some cases. Also, tough fibrous edema may be misinterpreted as obesity.

Other causes which are included in the causal list have similar mechanisms as mentioned in various other conditions. A few may have several mechanisms which are simultaneously effective. All this has the same line of treatment.

1. Medical treatment of underlying diseases
2. Diet management
3. Exercise
4. Maintenance of lost weight

Sometimes, being overweight is taken lightly, but looking at various serious conditions linked to it, timely management and treatment is very important.

Iatrogenic Obesity

Iatrogenic obesity is mainly pertaining to medicines taken for treatment of diabetes (insulin in particular) and some steroids.

Insulin Related Obesity

Several studies have proven a relationship between insulin treatment and weight gain. There have been studies where most of the diabetic patients gained weight over the study period in both arms, the insulin arm and Oral hypoglycemic agent arm, but patients taking insulin therapy gained weight very fast. The weight gain was significantly greater also. Across all therapies used in a study in UK, patients in the insulin treatment group gained on an average 4.0 kg more compared to patients in the conventional-treatment group.

This weight gain may be pertaining to better control on glucose levels; as suggested by glycosilated haemoglobin (HbA1C) levels between these two groups.

Ways to control diabetic treatment related obesity are:

1. *Lifestyle intervention:* Modify the lifestyle that suits diabetes and the recommended therapy. This in

particular includes restriction of fat and sugar in food and moderation and regularisation of the exercise.

2. Use of combination therapy: That is, a combination of oral drugs and insulin. For example, use of metformin as an insulin sensitiser.

3. Use of analogue insulin.

Steroid Related Obesity

Steroids, as discussed before are responsible for exogenic Cushing's syndrome. Yet, there are several reasons for steroid therapy:

1. Contraceptives: Hormonal oral contraceptive pills are steroidal in nature. Hence in some cases, they may lead to obesity.

2. Corticosteroid therapy as immunosuppressants: Steroid therapy as treatment for chronic conditions like autoimmune diseases, asthmatic bronchitis and certain cosmetic conditions.

These conditions involve steroid therapy for a long time which in turn leads to Cushing's disease and obesity.

Steroid related obesity is commonly seen without any medical need also. Many young boys misuse steroids for energy and body building while doing their exercises. There are several medical practitioners misusing steroids, especially in the lower socio-economic areas. These practices need to be controlled by being careful and asking the reason and possibility of avoiding it, especially if external steroids are prescribed in some cases. In case steroids are required, they should be properly tapered off before discontinuation and a balancing diet should be advised for nullifying their effect if any is highly important.

Malnutrition and Obesity

In developed countries, approximately 50 per cent or more cases pertain to malnutrition. The fact that the American population is almost pandemic to obesity is probably explained better on this ground.

Vitamin D Malnutrition and Obesity

Vitamin D is one of the major malnutrition types in obesity-causes. Let us recap a few facts:

1. Weight increases with higher latitudes and lower altitudes. The synthesis of vitamin D is known to be less in this geographic distribution. In fact, the latitude-altitude correlation does not apply to the

Arabic and Islamic population. This pertains to their custom of covering their skin, subsequently producing less vitamin D. As discussed earlier, they have a classical pattern of fat distribution also.

2. Weight increases in winters due to less vitamin D synthesis.

3. Genetic abnormalities with vitamin D deficiency is commonly associated with obesity.

4. Intake of vitamin D and calcium helps to burn fat.

5. Low (less than 25 IU) serum levels of vitamin D are associated with obesity. Higher vitamin D levels seem to have a positive effect on weight loss and sugar craving.

Vitamin D Therapy for Weight Loss

Vitamin D and calcium, when taken together are considered to be powerful fat burners. An European study has revealed that subjects with every 1 ng/ml increase in 25-hydroxycholecalciferol level in blood there is half pound more weight loss than diet control.

This therapy promotes early weight loss, but always needs a supporting calcium therapy as transaction of calcium is increased by vitamin D. Synthesis of vitamin D in sunlight is one of the ways of losing weight as well. Intake of vegetable vitamin D and calcium sources will help reduce weight as well. Intake of vitamin D by natural sources have high calorie content commonly, hence they should be taken with a conscious calorie management.

Other Malnutrition Related Obesity

Malnutrition of iron and 3-omega fatty acids is related to obesity. In many cases, some kinds of protein malnutrition conditions are also related with obesity. It is commonly seen that a diet rich in proteins helps reduce weight faster.

Deficiency of albumin in most of the cases is found related with increase in weight. Low vegetable diet and plant origin fats, along with low dietary fibers have an impact on weight gain, leading to increase in weight.

Proper diet management is required in cases where these conditions are in the background of obesity. Balanced diet with adequate intake of all micronutrients and conscious calorie management is very essential in this condition.

Malnutrition and Obesity: Review and Recap

1. Malnutrition of some types leads to obesity – this is the main cause of obesity in all developed countries.

2. Major malnutrition factors leading to obesity are – vitamin D deficiency, vitamin B complex deficiency (non-specific), 3-omega fatty acid deficiency, protein intake inadequacy – especially albumin and low dietary fibers.

3. Diet with low vegetable material with human intestinal microbes acting upon it, leads to obesity is experimented. Dietary fibers and plant origin fats are necessary parts of diet in a balanced diet.

4. Vitamin D and calcium intake effectively work as fat burners.

5. Vitamin D is synthesised by the skin in sunlight.

Chapter 5

Treatment of Obesity – Diet and Exercise

Treatment of obesity is infact management of weight and nutrition, and correction of any underlying defect. There are several algorithm plans for management of weight, but for the underlying medical conditions, only proper scientific medical treatment is the option. In this book, we have discussed many medical conditions linked with obesity and further we will discuss evaluation of obesity and associated symptoms for scientific, unbiased safe treatment of obesity.

Obesity and Underling Causes: Differential Diagnosis

For a proper evaluation, we will need a thorough recap of the previous chapters. There are various conditions discussed in depth in the previous chapters, which will help us understand the intensity of the underlying conditions of obesity. First, we rule out genetic diseases. If nothing else is found we reach the conclusion of metabolic obesity. The plan of action starts by noting down the history for ourselves, by asking questions listed below. Unbiased and honest answers to this questionnaire will lead us to a conclusion – the diagnosis. Once the diagnosis is established, we can help ourselves to manage weight.

Table 5.1 Questionnaire 1

When did I notice my obesity for the first time?	Childhood	Adolescence	Young adulthood (18-28)	Mid adulthood (28-40)	Adulthood (40+)
How did I confirm that I have obesity?	BMI / Weight monitoring	Waist size monitoring	Body fat analysis	Visual assessment	
Does anyone among my grandparents, parents and siblings have obesity?					
How is my exersion load? (Use the exercise calorie consumption chart as a guide)	Heavy physical exercise	Moderate physical exercise	Sedentary life with travelling	Sedentary life	Couch potato

(contd.)

How do I exercise?	Heavy	Moderate	Just a little	Nothing	Ristricted due to some condition
Do I eat/ snack just before bedtime?	Yes	No			
Which meals do I eat each day?	Breakfast	Lunch	Supper snacks	Dinner	Others
What and how much do I usually eat for breakfast?					
What and how much do I usually eat for lunch?					
What and how much do I usually eat for dinner?					
What are my favourite snacks?					
How much of them do I eat per sitting?					
Do I drink tea/ milk/ coffee as Pop up?	No	Yes			
How many servings per day?					
Do I drink juice?	No	Yes			
How much per day?					

(contd.)

(contd.)

How do I eat?	Overeat	Excessive snacking	Binge	Just to sateity	Less than satiety
How much alcohol do I take per week?	Nothing at all	30 ml	60 ml	120 ml	more than 120 ml
What pattern of obesity do I have?	Central apple pattern	Central pear pattern	General	Middle East pattern	Western pattern
Do I have any known conditions among the following:	Diabetes	Hypothyroidism	Genetic disorder	Eating disorder	Psychiatric disorder
How many times in a week do I eat or drink unjustifiedly?	Very often	Often	Not uncommon	Occasionally	Rarely

The second questionnaire Table 5.2 is more specific to rule out any underlying condition, if any, and to examine investigate and treat it completely. This questionnaire is rather a table to determine if you fit in any group of symptoms.

Table 5.2 Questionnaire 2

Sl. No.	Group of Symptoms Along with Obesity	Suspected Underlying Condition	Investigation(s)
1.	Frequency of thirst, hunger, frequent urination, especially at night, weakness and all gone feeling.	Diabetes mellitus	Fasting and post meal (2 hours) blood sugar estimation.

(contd.)

(contd.)

2.	Loss of memory, depression, dejection, constipation, loss of appetite, hoarseness of voice, fatigue, intolerance to cold, paleness, dryness and occasional itching of skin, muscle cramps/joint pains, slow pulse.	Hypothyroidism	Serum TSH, T3, T4 and free T4 evaluation.
3.	Increasing weight especially on face and abdomen, increased blood pressure, increased blood sugar, pimples on face or recent origin, fat deposition on shoulder, collar bone, excessive sweating, thinning reddish-bluish discolouration of the skin, loss of sleep, loss of libido, euphoria or depression.	Cushing's syndrome	ACTH and cortisol evaluation, especially if suppressed by dexamethasone.
4.	Small head, strabismus, high and narrow palate, small jaw, mouth almost always open, high nasal bridge, polydactyl, down slanting eyes, tapered and short figures — all are congenital.	Cohen's syndrome	Diagnosis is usually clinical and will be made by a very early age.

(contd.)

(contd.)

5.	Recurrent, episode-wise binge eating, feeling that he cannot control eating in an episode, eating a larger amount, eating in discreet periods, reflex compensatory behaviour (usually to induce weight loss), use of laxative purgatives without medical advice.	Eating disorder	Psychological counselling
6.	Muscle pain, weak bones/fractures, low energy/constant fatigue, low immunity (getting sick often), depression or mood swings, irregular sleeping patterns.	Vitamin D low	Vitamin D level

The above six conditions are the most commonly detectable conditions which lead to immediate complications in obesity. This does not mean that once these six conditions are excluded, there is no complication or risk, and all the underlying conditions are ruled out. But in most cases, after the exclusion of the above six conditions, metabolic obesity is the only remaining cause left. Now, when we are clear about how obesity appears, we can proceed for the treatment of obesity.

General Considerations for the Treatment of Obesity

As mentioned above, treatment of obesity includes:

1. Medicinal treatment, especially for the underlying cause
2. Diet management
3. Exercise
4. Avoiding complication and maintaining the lost weight
5. Counselling in almost all cases

Medicinal management of obesity includes two considerations:

1. Treatment of the underlying cause, especially if there is any emergency to be addressed.
2. Treatment of the already present complications.
3. Treatment for weight loss.

There are several modes of treatment available in various systems of medicine and paramedical sciences.

We consider here the same in two groups. Primary group is the compulsory part of obesity treatment – diet, exercise and muscle training, and the secondary group is medication. Medication is further divisible as medication for losing weight and medication for the underlying cause. The Fig. 5.1 below explains the most applicable plan of treatment:

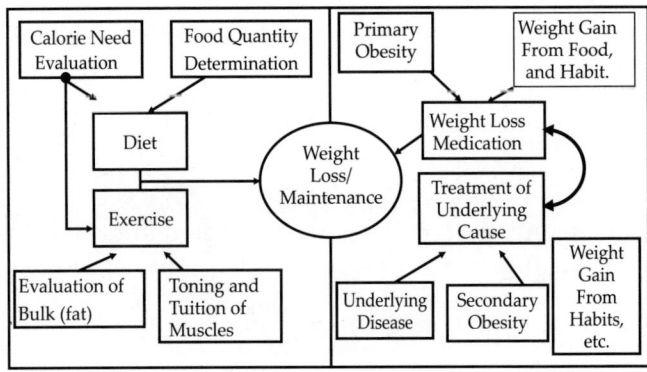

Fig. 5.1 Plan of Treatment

Getting started with the treatment of obesity –

1. Measure, evaluate, access the excess weight – Rule out medical conditions.
2. Understand the contribution of fat in the weight – from percentage body fat analysis.
3. Determine the goal of weight to be reduced.
4. Determine the period over which the weight is to be lost.
5. Collect inputs for planning, such as – how much time can you spend for exercise.

6. Plan for a weight loss program.

7. Make up your mind.

8. Start.

9. Maintain a diary or chart for monitoring weight vs diet.

10. Review every three weeks.

Measure, Evaluate, Access the Excess Weight – Rule Out Medical Conditions

To start with a workable weight loss plan, like any other task aimed, we need to set a few prerequisites. Therefore, the first step is to determine what is to be achieved. Do I need to lose weight? If yes, how much weight should I lose? From where do I gain this weight? Do I have any underful medical condition, etc. This will lead to a thorough evaluation of the status of obesity.

Measure – the first few things to measure are weight, height, belly height or weight circumference, chest circumference, neck circumference and skin fold thicknesses.

Calculate BMI from the formulae stated above and now compare your height, weight and BMI with standards to know whether you need to lose weight and can you afford to lose weight We have asked ourselves a second question, pertaining to the next data which is likely to add a desire to lose some pounds– the waist circumference or the belly height. In many people, there is a central pattern of obesity, with weight within normal range but high abdominal fat. In such conditions, for medical and cosmetic reasons, weight loss may be a desirable act.

Anyway, once it is decided how much weight we need to and afford to lose, we continue evaluating the next parameter – belly height/waist circumference. Higher weight circumference may have cosmetic, and sometimes obesity related risk problems. For this reason, one has to know if there is a necessity for reduction of this circumference.

We also keep the data from various other measurements ready and the calculations done. Evaluation of a few medical underlying conditions, especially if there is any point of the second questionnaire is very important. Carefully rule out any underlying medical cause, with medical help. This is critically important before we go for further management of obesity. We also keep a data of cholesterol, haemoglobin, serum calcium levels and blood glucose levels (fasting) for future reference.

Now, at the end of this stage we have the following inputs ready with which we can proceed to the next stage in the plan.

- Am I obese or overweight? – Yes / No
  - If yes, how have I decided – visually or by weight and height proportion study
- Do I need to lose weight? Yes / No
  - If yes – how much (to bring the BMI at 20)
  - If no – do I feel I should lose weight (such as due to high abdominal fat / medical reasons/ others)? Yes/ No
    - If yes, do I afford to lose weight? Yes/ No
      - If yes, how much?
    - If no, how do I manage to maintain myself to a fit figure?
- Do I have a medical condition to be treated? Yes/ No
  - If yes – consult the doctor
  - If no – proceed for further steps

Understand the Contribution of Fat in the Weight – From Percentage Body Fat Analysis

Once we have considered the evaluation of the losable weight, we have to understand the source of this excess weight, if any. We have formulae for calculations as in chapter 1. In the previous step, we have measured certain additional statistics. The skin fold thickness and neck circumference should be used to estimate body fat percentage. Calculation of body fat percentage will help us understand how much fat is to be burnt in all.

For example, consider the following chart:

Height in cms	165
Current weight (A)	68
BMI	25
Ideal maximum weight (B)	59.90
Weight to be lost (A-B)	8.11
Energy required daily	2352.5
Energy gained daily	2392.00
Energy to be lost daily	2080.28
Period for loss of weight (days)	30
Daily intake of energy	1413.71
Energy to be generated from body fats	938.79

Skin fold area	thickness in mm
Pectoral	25
Mid-axillary	25
Suprailiac (lateral abdominal)	37.5
Abdominal	62.5
Thigh	25
On the shoulder blade apex	18.75
Back of the arm	20
Sum thickness of the skin folds	213.75
Gender factor constant 1	0.0008267
Age	33

Energy to be lost by daily	0.00
Total body fat	3299.29
Average essential body fat (percentage)	2.50
Losable fat (percentag)	46.02
Losable fat (grams)	3129.29

Gender factor constant 2	0.00012828
Body mass density	0.94164551
Body fat percentage (formula skin fold)	75.68
Body fat percentage (formula BMI)	21.36
Average	48.52

From this sheet, it is clear that the person's BMI, fat under multiple deposition area and type of food taken impact the losable weight. In this case, it is also clear that even if the BMI-wise moderate weight does not suggest much weight loss, the weight loss is strongly suggested by the body's fat percentage. This stage gives us an exact idea as to how much is to be lost exactly and how much do we need to lose from fats stored in the body.

The formula also suggests – as quickly as one wants to lose weight, one needs to lose it from fat stores, whereas the loss in weight is more in form of loss of energy if the time taken is longer.

Setting the Goal of Weight to be Lost

The goal of weight to be lost is set from the above calculations, depending upon one's diet, use of energy and disposition to store fats. What we tend to lose more is, in particular, the below skin fat of the body.

The Period for Losing the Weight

The weight loss period is determined from two factors:

1. Why are we losing the fat? – medical reason / cosmetic reason
2. How much (mainly physique-wise) energy expenditure is possible by exercise?

One very important point to be noted is – shorter the period of weight loss, higher the loss of body fat. This brings upon few risk factors – medical as well as cosmetic. Also, quickly lost fat recovers quicker. Hence, unless medical emergencies such as high cardiac risk prevail, no one should opt an option of weight loss in quicker time.

Ideal period for weight loss is fractioned into two – rapid weight loss – 45 per cent of the total weight to be lost and slow 65 per cent of the total weight to be lost. The method of calculation is given as follows.

Total weight to be Lost	5 kgs	
45 per cent for rapid loss		15 days
65 per cent for slow loss	2.25	51 days
Total period	3.25	66 days

The weight period should be 25 per cent for first 45 per cent of weight loss and 75 per cent of the time for next 65 per cent. This is calculated at rate of 0.15 kg per day, approximately during rapid weight loss and 0.1 kg per day during slow weight loss. At the end of phase I, calculations must be repeated.

Information collected from questionnaire:

This will give us a fair idea regarding things which play an important role in weight loss plan.

- How much time am I sincerely willing to give for my exercise?
- How much do I need to eat to feel satisfied?
- Which food I cannot leave or not control?
- What food can I easily jeopardise?
- How much sugar / fructose can I avoid from the current scenario?

The answers of all these questions are available even before we started to speak of planning, from the questionnaire, to keep the mind unbiased. All these answers now form a basis for planning.

Planning for the Weight Loss Programme

Planning for weight loss includes three parts:

1. Diet
2. Exercise
3. Counselling (self and external)

Table 5.3 Diet – Balanced vs Obesity Control Diet Program

Head	Balanced Diet	Weight Management Program
Components	Macronutrients: Fats, carbohydrates, proteins in acceptable macronutrient disbursement range. Fibers in food in an adequate amount.	Proteins are major diet factors. Depending upon dietary needs and plan, carbohydrates and fibers quality is adjusted. Facts are restricted as much as possible.
	Micronutrients: All vitamins in adequate quantity, emphasis on the natural sources of vitamins and minerals.	Micronutrients: All vitamins in adequate quantity with slightly higher vitamin D; emphasis on natural sources of vitamins and minerals.

(contd.)

(contd.)

Sugars	Free and fruit sugars as required.	Free sugars – low; highly restricted fruit sugars.
Quantity	As per required to achieve satiety.	Calories to be matched, rest of the calories to be filled in by fillers.
Animal food	Allowed animal food as a component.	Animal food is restricted. Only increase if there is no substitute for animal foods available, few low fat animal food like milk and dairy products can be allowed.
Alcohol	Permitted in low quantities.	No alcohol allowed.

Characteristics of a balanced Diet

The diet should include all components of the complete nutrition profile as discussed in nutrition and obesity.

1. It should form enough bulk of food to satisfy the person's hunger.
2. The energy derived from each component should be within the agreed range.
3. It should have enough calories to meet the person's daily requirements.

Modification of a Balanced Diet for Weight Management

Weight management diet is more of an individual effort depending upon one's food habits, likings, requirement, work and exercise. Yet, for reducing weight, there are a few principles of diet management listed below:

1. Do not starve, keep your diet full in quantity as required by your stomach.
2. Consume low energy foods. Use more fillers to build quantity. These fillers are generally fibers.
3. Maintain minimum adequate energy intake of carbohydrates, reduce fats to almost zero.
4. Maintain adequate protein intake.
5. Maintain adequate intake of micronutrients – vitamins and minerals.
6. Take enough water.
7. Use more vegetable than cereals.
8. No animal origin food should be consumed.
9. No alcohol.

Weight Reduction Diet – Control Program

Weight reduction diet is not a one-time planning; it is a complete programmed arrangement for staged weight loss. This program has various stages depending upon the dietician need of the patient and associated factors. The standard weight loss diet can be designed in four stages:

1. Rapid weight loss
2. Slower, stable weight loss
3. Maintained low weight
4. Adaptation to the controlled diet for correct weight

Each of this stage works the best when properly organised and target oriented. Before actually starting to diet, the target of each stage must be well set. This target is set on the following credentials:

1. How much ideal weight is to be lost? (How much weight will bring one to the upper limit of the normal BMI range?)
2. How much fasting does the person's work-load profile afford?
3. What is the role of exercise in the current scenario? Is the same going to continue or are you planning to modify?

Depending upon these credentials, a diet is planned in such a way that the person's calorie requirement calculatedly is met, without compromise to his intake in quantity and taste. This elaborate information is systematically assembled as a flow chart, as follows.

1. Weight to be lost as predetermined and calculated*1 → Weight driven from excessive body fat → Exercise suggested/done → Quantity required per day → Adjust the food.
2. Quantity required from daily habit → Amount of calories to be consumed to reduce weight to target*2 → Design the food with the calories required derived from carbohydrates mostly and strictly calculating the non-sensible and sensible fat*3 → Add all micronutrients and tasty spices → Use fibers as fillers (roughage and leafy vegetables).
3. Maintain protein quantity required per day → Sprouted pulses and milk → Avoid food of animal origin.

Principles of a Feasible and Long-lasting Diet Program

1. Do not remain hungry — help yourself, satisfy your hunger fully — with exponentially reduced quantity — fill in the diet with fibers.

---

*1 => Weight to be lost = current weight – weight for BMI set at 23 (for rapid) to 20 (slower)

*2 => Calories to be burnt = body's current excess fat (weight to be lost in kilo's) x calories per kilo of body fat (7700)

*3 => Non-sensible fat-fat intake in the form of milk, fructose; fruit, nut, vegetable ingredients, etc.
Sensible fat - fat used for frying, deep frying, seasoning, dressing and garnishing.

This can happen in the following manner:

As calculated, the diet food should be adjusted to the calories required per day. This food is based upon the principle of adequate macronutrient and micronutrient sources and their requirement positioned well. Once this builds its quantity, we add some calorie-free/very low calorie fillers. These fillers are mainly fibers and roughages like leafy vegetables, husk of wheat ground, sprouts, etc. They should be used as fillers in food. Basically, the diet plan should be determined in a conjugate manner. For example, if a vegetable is being cooked, it should contain a good amount of leafy vegetables and vegetables should not be peeled.

Also, cereals and supportive should be well designed and planned, as will be discussed further in details. This whole exercise revolves around two facts:

i. Determination, set mind and firm decision.
ii. Getting a balanced and calorie restricted diet.

2. Do not compel perversion of regular seasoning/spices/taste unless extremely required – learn cooking without oil instead.

Seasoning has no additional calories of itself. Unless the seasoning is added with fat, there is no harm in taking the seasoning or spices. These seasonings add taste to the food. When we plan for a diet control, we have to restrict energy and not the taste. Maintaining taste and quantity of your food, usually becomes an additional incentive to continue with the restricted diet. Loss of regular taste and quantity, in contrast, many times limits the determination. There are three steps of supporting the diet program:

i. *Use your regular seasoning* – the way you like it, but refrain from oil, cream and any other type of fat and cheese.

ii. *Learn to cook without oil* – this can be achieved by roasting your spices instead of frying them in oil. Use of teflon coated non-stick cookware is good for this purpose. Immediately after the minimal toasting of spices is over, add a small quantum of water to it so that the spices are well cooked. Also boiled/cooked vegetable will make the food taste as your regular food.

iii. *Spices and seasonings do not have their own calories* – considering this fact, we can keep some powdered seasoning handy and add it on top of the food. This will add to your familiar taste of food and will not make you remember or think of your regular food. It will also keep you from getting discouraged by your diet plan.

The moral of the story is – let your diet plan not become a burden but let it be as comfortable as your regular diet.

3. Boost your mind for refraining from over eating and eating between meals – help yourself by keeping busy.

   This step is probably the peak of your patience test, especially for early diet controllers; this is the most critical requisite. Usually excess energy is consumed by poping snacks. These snacks are highly energy rich, non-nutritious foods. This food is eaten more as a psychological factor, than being a requirement or hunger-driven desire.

   For being prudent on this matter, observe the trend of your pop-up eating time, condition and circumstance. Avoid getting into this trend by keeping yourself busy at that time, place and circumstance. You have already identified your favourite snacks. Avoid getting these snacks in your office, home and wherever we can go on hogging it.

4. If at all your balance of calorie intake is lost, determinedly adjust it in the successive meals.

Still in some cases, there are possibilities where you end up eating more than the regular controlled diet. Just calculate the excess energy intake. Once you know the excess energy intake, adjust your next meals in such a way that you take in less energy. This will average your energy requirements in three meals.

Planning a diet starts with the calculation of your energy and quantity requirements – as we have done by answering questionnaire 1. Further in this chapter, we also have a chart where minute-wise energy consumption for all activities is jotted down. Combining the questionnaire with this chart will help, you in managing energy intake versus expenditure besides calculating energy planning well.

Component Wise Impact of Stages of Weight Loss on Food

There is some energy profile specific to all macronutrients. This profile determines if the macronutrient is supposed to be deposited in body. Fat and carbohydrates are stored in the body. Proteins stay in equilibrium. In the absence of glucoses, derivations from, carbohydrates and proteins are used for glyconeogensis that is, production of glucose within the body. Hence, an adequate amount of carbohydrates, more amounts of proteins and a restriction of fats is usually the key of diet planning.

Table 5.4 Stages of Weight-loss Planning

Stage 1	Stage 2	Stage 3	Stage 4
Rapid Weight Loss	Slow and Steady Weight Loss	Maintaining Low Weight	Adoption of a Newly Designed Diet
4th day of dieting to 90th day of dieting. But this period can vary depending upon calculations as discussed earlier.	91st to 120th day of dieting.	120th to 180th day of dieting.	Sustained from 90 days to 300 days.
Restriction of fat (0.15 g/kg body weight) – all this fat is derived out of insensible fats – no free fat should be taken in.	Restriction of fat (0.3 g/kg body weight) – maximum 0.1 gm/kg body weight should be driven out of sensible fat.	Restriction of fat (0.4 g/kg body weight).	Optimally lowest fat (0.3 g/kg body weight).
Increased (maximum) fiber.	Optimum quantity of fibers (sprouts, vegetables, fruits, all other roughage).	Reducing fiber quantity gradually.	Good amount of fibers.
Lowest optimum carbohydrates (2.5 – 3 g/kg body weight).	Optimum carbohydrates (3– 4 g/kg body weight).	Optimum (no change) carbohydrates.	Optimum (no change) carbohydrates.

(contd.)

(contd.)

Protein quantity a bit increased, micronutrients and water quantity – unchanged.	Protein increased up to 1.5 g/kg body weight, micronutrients and water quantity – unchanged.	Proteins – managed (1.5 – 2 g/kg body weight)	No further change in proteins.
		Water increased	Increased water intake.
Diet balanced in micronutrients and modified for carbohydrates and fat. This intake of carbohydrates will be dependent on how much weight is to be lost.		Micronutrients – unchanged	Micronutrients – unchanged

Individual Diet Design

Inputs:

Current weight

Weight to be lost

Body fat percentage

Calories required per day as calculated

Calories to be lost

Amount of calories to be produced from body fats

Calculations of Macronutrients for Stage 1

Fat quantity QF = Current body weight × 0.15 gm

Calories from fat CF = QF × 9 calories

Carbohydrates range QCH = Current body weight × 2.5 – current body weight × 3

Calories from CHO C CHO = Calories from carbohydrates max × 4 calories

Amount of proteins QP = [Required calories – (CF + CHO + 4 gm

Amount of fillers (such as salads, green vegetables, fruits) = Quantity required – quantity built by macronutrients in case the fruits have a lot of sugar content, their 2/3 should be calculated under carbohydrates.

Required fibers = Required quantity of food – (QF + QCHO + QP)

> QF = Fat quantity
> CF = Calories from fat
> QCH = Quantity of carbohydrates
> QCHO = Calories from carbohydrates

Care to be taken while designing a diet plan:

1. Do not reduce carbohydrate income lower than lower limit of AMDR.
2. Do not reduce protein intake less than AMDR.
3. Replace fat to fat free (restriction of sensible fat).

4. Restrict use of sugar containing beverages and diet. Stop alcoholic beverages.

As a general guide, for losing weight, the following formula may also be used for calculation of nutrients per day. This should constitute approximately – 2300 calories energy per day even for a sedentary lifestyle.

- Carbohydrates → 4 – 4.4 gm/kg body weight/per day
- Protein → 1.6 - 2 gm/kg body weight/per day
- Fat → 0.2 - 0.6 gm/kg body weight/per day

Anything required above this quantity should be a fiber or roughage to be had as a filler. Say for example, for a 90 kg body:

- Carbohydrates – 360 gm (1440)
- Protein – 180 gm (720)
- Fats – 54 gm (486)
- Total energy food – 600 gm – calories 2600
- If someone is habitual of eating larger quantities, roughage should be filled in for the rest of the quantity. In this calculation, the amount of fat, carbohydrates and proteins in leaves, cereals, sprouts, curd, spices, vegetables, pods, nuts, fruits, sugars, beverages, everything must be considered while calculating.

Some additional tips for the diet plan:

i. Use honey in place of sugar wherever possible.

ii. Replace rice and wheat by jawar (sorghum) as and where possible.
iii. Use fresh food instead of canned or stale food.
iv. Avoid using too much salt, seasoning and spices in the food or regular cooking.

For example:	Desired weight:
Current weight: 85 kg	64 kgs (height – 167 cm)
Weight to be lost: 21 kg	Quantity taken per day: 2270
Calories required: 2248 calories	

Design

Body weight 85 kg   Food quantity required 2270   Energy required 2248

Table 5.5 Typical Changes from Balanced Diet to Low Energy Balanced Diet

		Current Food Intake			Planned Intake			
	Contributor	Quantity	Energy	Per Kg BW	Quantity	Energy	Per Kg BW	Quantity Planned
Carbohydrates	Chappati	700	2800	14.529	147	588	3.61	212.5
	Rice	200	800		42	168		
	Other cereals	10	40		2.1	8.4		
	Sugars/Beverages	25	100		5.25	21		
	Fruits	50	200		10.5	42		
	Milk (1 l = 1050 gms)	250	310		100	124		

(contd.)

		Current Food Intake			Planned Intake			
	Contributor	Quantity	Energy	Per Kg BW	Quantity	Energy	Per Kg BW	Quantity Planned
Proteins	Pulses and sprouts (including idly, pasta)	100	400	6.2353	59	236	1.9435294	307.725
	Animal non-milk protein	0	0		0	0		
	Milk	250	280			244		
	Milk proteins (chasin, etc)	25	100		14.75	59		
	Eggs		0		0	0		
	Salads / Vegetables	100	300		59	177		
	Fruits	50	100		29.5	118		
	Others (like 5 percent of rice, 0.3 percent of wheat)	5	20		2.95	11.8		
Fats	Free (cream, cheese, oil, fat, ghee, butter)	20	180	0.6471	0	0	0.0270588	12.75
	In vegetable curries	25	225		0	0		
	In non-vegetarian curries		0		0	0		
	Unsensible	10	90		2.3	20.7		
	Animal food		0		0	0		
	Milk		225		0	45		
	Fruits		90		0	0		
Fibers / Fillers		400	50		1745.65	436.41		
		2220	6110		474.35	2299.3		532.975

Taking this basic calculation into consideration, we can refine and define the diet plan for the person. Add vitamin D and calcium to the diet if required. The protein quantity can be added to it if the AMDR is not achieved while planning by energy (as is the case in this chart). But this should be carefully managed as shown in the chart above. The diet of the person looks to be carb-dominated as the salads / vegetable quantity is less. Milk quantity per day should be restricted. Moreover, milk should be skimmed to remove all possible fat from it. As there is a little scope for reduction of fat for restricting energy, sugars and fruits with high sugar will be the next targets. In many cases, the calories taken may not be correctly monitored. Hence, before the next step of energy expenditure planning, at least for ten days, a well monitored diet setting is required. This is possible after complete clarity about intake and expenditure of energy is established.

An important point likely to be missed in this whole exercise is adequate vitamin and mineral intake management. While planning for raw food material and articles in vegetable food or spices, enough amounts of vitamin sources should be given a proper place. The same matter should be considered with minerals. In Appendix II, common salad and food articles along with their calories and nutrition contents are listed. The appendix can be referred to for this purpose.

Planning Exercise for Obesity

For the effort of weight reduction, exercise is an inevitable factor. A series of exercises are very important for burning calories. Energy is always lost in any form of physical activity. Depending upon one's weight, daily activities lose some amount of energy from the body. Phase II is state to set your "wet set Point" hence careful calculation of intake and expenditure of energy is vitally important before the step starts.

The chart below is an approximate calculation of calorie use in exercise per hour. For all calculations of weight dependent calorie loss, these activities shouls be taken into considerations as per their contribution in one's daily timetable.

Table 5.6 Energy Consumed per hour in Routine Activities and Excercises

Daily Activity		Gardening /Additional Activity		Sports		Dancing / Breathing Exercise	
Sleeping	55	Digging	500	Golf with trolley	180	Studio / Classical	650
Eating	85	Hoeing	350	Golf without trolley	240	Aerobic/ Cardio	420
Sitting	85	Planting	250	Hiking	500	Ballroom	260
Standing	100	Knitting	85	Jogging, 5 mph	500	Skating	420
Driving	110	Sewing	85	Step aerobics	550	Cross country ski machine	500
Office work	140	Power walking	600	Swimming, active	500	Pranayam	100
House-work-moderate	160	Bicycling, moderate	450	Table tennis	290	Kapal bhati	280

Walking	280		Tennis	350	Bhasrika	300
Bathing, massaging, etc.	130		Water aerobics	400	Yoga asana	530
			Power walking	600	Surya namaskar	550
			Rowing	550	Meditation/ Chanting	55
			Running	700		
			Jogging	500		

The exercise needs to be designed according to the exertion profile, weight to be lost, time frame, disposition of the person etc. All excess fat is burnt from exercise. The fundamental principle of weight loss is restricting weight gain from restriction of intake of storable energy and burning any and all stored energy by exercise. All the energy present in the body in the form of fat will be lost by daily activity in case of a completely fat restricted diet. If there is a fat/potential fat intake out of proportion, there cannot be any balance between lost calories and consumed calories. All excess fat stores need to be lost by exercise. Hence, in obese cases, the energy equation has three variables – the current energy intake, the required energy intake and energy to be generated from stored fat. For calculation of energy to be lost from stored fat, we use body fat percentage and absolute fat mass.

Let us consider a scenario:

Sex	Male
Height in cms	165
Current weight (A)	85
BMI	31
Ideal maximum weight (B)	59.90
Weight to be lost (A-B)	25.1
Energy required daily	2352.5
Energy gained daily	4334.00
Energy to be lost daily	1610.90
Period for loss of weight (days)	120
Energy to be intaken daily	2014.49

Skin fold area	Thickness in mm
Pectoral	32.5
Mid-axillary	27.5
Suprailliac (lateral abdominal)	40
Abdominal	67.5
Thigh	27.5
On the shoulder blade apex	18.75
Back of the arm	20
Sum thickness of the skin folds	233.75
Gender factor constant 1	0.0008267

Energy to be generated from body fats	338.01
Energy to be lost by exercise daily	1046.62
Total body fat	4719.33

Age	33
Gender factor constant 2	0.00012828
Body mass density	0.93012351

Average essential body fat (percentage)	2.50
Losable fat (percentage)	53.02
Losable fat in gms	4506.83

Body fat percentage (formula skin fold)	82.19
Body fat percentage (formula BMI)	28.86
Average	55.52

Here, depending upon one's weight, period required to lose energy and body's fat percentage, approximately 1100 kcal energy needs to be lost by the person from exercise. This statement is to propose that simple exercises are not enough for weight loss, but may have different purposes. Hence energy components must be considered while programming exercises for weight loss there are exercises with various purposes. Usually rapid exercise is for building cardiac and pulmonary capacity. Hence, a well planned exercise is very important. Moreover the coordination of diet and exercise also needs to be reviewed.

The Table 5.7 below has a coordinate bond of exercise and stage of dieting

Table 5.7

Stage	Stage 1	Stage 2	Stage 3	Stage 4
Phase	Rapid weight loss	Slow steady weight loss	Maintaining low weight	Adoption of newly designed diet
Tenure	First 25 per cent time of day of dieting.	Next 75 per cent time period of day of dieting.	120th to 180th day.	Sustained from 90 days to 300 days.
Role of carbohydrates	Maintain-quick nutrition, mainly body metabolism.	Maintenance of BMI, major quick nutrition, prevention of starvation.	Maintenance of body's BMR and regular energy supply.	Regular body nutrition share (restored to normal).
Role of Protein	Body maintenance, as catabolism is very high, emergency energy source if required.	Reconstruction, prevention of damage, muscle building.	Regular reformations and reconstructions (restored to regular function).	Restored to regular function.

(contd.)

(contd.)

Role of fat	Lubrication of joints, skin and moving muscles.	Lubrication of joints, skin and moving muscles, supplement for hormone synthesis, cholesterol, etc.	Contribution to the energy profile of the body, increasing fat tolerance, supporting proteins in shaping and tuition of muscles.	Restored to regular function.
Exercise	Slow, graduating to high moderate but not too fast (protocol 1).	Stable at high moderate	Stable at moderate to slow moderate (protocol 3) + muscle tuition.	Slow moderate or regular exertion profile
Role of Exercise	Consumption of all excess daily calorie intake.	(protocol 2) + muscle tuition.	Restriction of weight gain.	(muscle tuition).
		Consumption of calories to equate intake.		Almost none if not doing any special exercise.

(contd.)

This chart speaks of the exercise protocols. The protocols are stated below. Basically, for all stages of exercise, various speed quantum and person's capacity and expertise of doing an exercise are included in the protocols. The willingness for the exercise may be one of the factors, which probably has been considered in making these protocols, hence various options are available. Even if these protocols are not complete, they are guidelines for one, who is trying to design his diet and exercise plan.

Usually, people start with exercising suddenly and then suddenly stopping. This may lead to certain complaints and increase tendency of the body for storing fats. Another error is rapidly raising the speed of exercise, which may make muscles stiff, their shape are molded and increase weight loss time. Ideal exercise should be started slowly, so that very small amount of carbohydrates are broken down and fat breakdown is stimulated. Once, in approximately 6-8 minutes, the fat breakdown starts and the carbohydrate energy consumption is minimised, rapid exercise should be done till one is exhausted with the energy. This exhaustion indicates that all excess glucose/glycogen in the muscles and all ready energy is over. After this, regeneration of glucose by glyconeogensesis is required, so slow recovering and synchronising relaxation is required. The exercise, in this way, will help burn fat to the maximum. All these protocols are designed for approximately one hour. They can be modified according to the requirement of energy loss and the time available.

Exercise Programs for Weight Reduction

Table 5.7 Protocol 1

Time From Start	Purpose	Breathing Exercise	Modern Exercise	Dancing Exercises	Yoga	Walk	Gymnastics
0 - 9 minutes	Warm up	Pranayam, kapalbhati.	Round up motions	Feet and arms	Shavasan, lying	Slow, normal walk (2 -3 kmph) 2 - 3 rounds.	Climbing up, hanging, inversion.
10 - 15 minutes	Escalation	Rapid kapalbhati, bhas-rika.	Rapid round up of multiple joints and organs, touching toes with crossing arms.	Legs, arms, chest	Sitting exer-cises	Fast walk 2 rounds (2.5 -3 km/ph).	Simple Double bar exercises.
16 - 45 minutes	Peak exercise	Rapid kapalbhati, bhasrika and rechak.	Very rapid exercise, sit ups, cardio exercise.	Legs, arms, chest, belly, neck, head.	Standing exercises, inversions, Surya namaskar.	Jogging (4 -4.5 kmph); Running (5-6.5 kmph).	Rapid double bar exercises + single par exercises + hanging and lifting exercises.

(contd.)

(contd.)

| 46 - 50 min | Recovery. | Pranayam, normal breathing. | Lying down and vibration. | Legs | Shavasan | Very slow Walk | Partial hanging |

Table 5.8 Protocol 2

Time From Start	Purpose	Breathing Exercise	Modern Exercise	Dancing Exercises	Yoga	Walk	Gymnastics
0-20 minutes	Warm up and reformation.	Pranayam and slow kapalbhati.	Rounding motions and slow progressive movements.	Feet and legs, arms motion.	Lying and sitting exercises.	Slow walk 1 round, 3-4 rounds fast walk.	Single and double bar exercise.
21- 40 minutes	Maintenance of energy state.	Rapid kapalbhati and rechak.	Fast sustained movements of body parts.	slow aerobic/ ball	Standing and stretching exercises.	Jogging	Double bar exercise.
41- 45 min	Recovery	Pranayam.	Stretch and relax	Feet and legs, arms in motion.	Sitting relaxation, savasana.	Standing with hands on knees.	Partial inversion.

Table 5.9 Protocol 3

Time From Start	Purpose	Breathing Exercise	Modern Exercise	Dancing Exercises	Yoga	Walk	Gymnastics
0-30 minutes	Warm up and reformation.	Pranayam and slow kapalbhati.	Slow and gradually increasing exercise of arms and all small joints.	Feet and leg, arms motion.	Lying and sitting exercises.	Slow walk 1 round, 3-4 rounds fast walk.	Single and double bar exercise.
31-40 min	Maintenance of energy state.	Rechak and mild kapalbhati.	Fast, sustained movement of body parts.	Slow aerobic/ball.	Standing and stretching exercises.	Jogging	Double bar exercise.
41-45 minutes	Recovery	Pranayam	Stretch and relax.	Feet and legs, arms motion.	Sitting relaxation, savasana.	Standing with hands on knees.	Sitting relaxed

Muscle Tuition

Muscle tuition is an exercise especially to build the shape and restrict fats from depositing into the looser area. This will benefit almost 60 percent population practicing it. Muscle tution is available in various forms. It can be tight ligature with long cloth or readymade as available in the market with periodical compressions and vibrations. The basic logic of this effort is to burn out the fat and help body occupy the loose tissue with non-adipose tissue, especially muscles. Muscles also are toned and shaped in by this depending upon the technique used.

Technique 1

Binding with the cloth: this should be done immediately following the recovery stages of all protocols.

The rules:

1. The cloth should be absorbent, of cotton or linen – a thin cloth.
2. The direction of wrapping should be from down to up in overlapping spikes, covering entire belly.
3. Its wrapping should be as tight as tolerable.
4. For abdominal wrapping, wrap on a deep expiration evacuated belly.
5. On the chest, the wrapping is only for breast support and elevation.

The duration of wrapping should vary according to the organ, tolerance and comfort. For abdomen, it can be left even overnight.

Technique 2

Vibrating Belt: This belt is available in the market. It produces periodical, smooth and coarse vibrations. This belt is worn across the organ at its maximum muscle bulk and can be set on various speeds depending upon tolerance. This will help in tuning the muscles and in giving them shape.

The belt works by producing vibrations in the muscle bulk. This belt is also programmed to create periodical compression and relaxation of the muscle bulk. This also leads to virtual exercise of the muscle. Due to this, there is consumption of fats and reformation of muscle bulk. This gives a shape and burns extra fat out of the part it is exposed to.

Technique 3

Sauna Belts: Sauna belt is a heat function combined belt with compression. The fat in the tired muscles is catabolised rapidly for energy consumption, in the presence of compression and heat. This promotes early loss of bulk. This will be an additional risk for tanning of skin in some cases, hence be careful.

A good weight loss program is an orchestra of diet, exercise and muscle tuition. All these three factors can even individually aid to reduce weight to a large extent, but all three together help making a healthy profile.

Psychological and medical reasons are also prevalent behind obesity for which immediate action is required.

Technique 4

Massage: Massages for muscle tuition is a famous traditional way. The muscles should be rapidly massaged and irritated by hands, with the help of oil or water. The areas where massage is required are:

1. Abdomen
2. Buttocks
3. Back, as far as the arms can reach
4. All other fat deposit areas
5. Thighs and knees

Muscle tuition in this method is by rapid hand movements on the area. This massage is preferably performed in both or from down to up motions. The steps for massage with oil in a lying down position are:

1. Apply oil over the skin and the area to be massaged.
2. Rapidly move the hands, the palms all over the area, from all sides.
3. Continue the massage till the area feels fully irritated.

4. After this, the area is tightly tied or held in till it relaxes. This gives the best results.

Massage for muscle tuition is also advised while bathing. It can be done under a shower or on a wet body, with (even soap can act as a lubricant) or without lubricants; the massage should be done in the same way as with oil. After this a lot of water should be poured over the part, which is then tightly drawn in by the force of stretch.

Massage can also be done with the force of flowing water. Blunt but a forceful stream of water should strike against the area intended to be massaged, and massage should be done with the force of water.

Review and Recap

1. Treatment of obesity is rather management of weight and nutrition, and correction of any underlying defect.
2. Weight to be lost and period in which weight is to be lost should be set well before we start the plan. This will also include calculation of various other parameters.

3. An ideal diet for weight control is a modified balanced diet with all micronutrients and macronutrients in the following manner:

    a. Carbohydrates: 4-4.4 gm/kg body weight/day
    b. Protein: 1.6-2 gms/kg body weight/day.
    c. Fat: 0.2-0.6 gms/kg body weight/day.

4. Exercise for weight loss has multiple protocols, starting all and ending slowly and reaching a peak which will help reduce the fat adequately in adequate time.

5. The fundamental principle of weight loss is restricting weight gain from restriction of intake of storable energy and burning any and all stored energy by exercise.

6. There are four ways of muscles tuition, the third component of treatment of weight reduction:

    a. Tying by cloth
    b. Sauna belt
    c. Vibrating belt
    d. Massage

    i. Oil massage

    ii. Water stream massage

    iii. Massage while bathing

7. Starvation, losing taste in your routine food and fasting for your favourite seasoning/Spices is discouraged. Doing so will increase the chances of losing determination.

Chapter 6

Treatment of Obesity – Medicinal Therapy

Obesity and Medicinal Therapy

The medicinal therapy for obesity includes two aspects:

1. The treatment of its underlying cause
2. Treatment specific to weight loss

Various systems of medicine have different approaches to obesity medication.

Allopathic Medicine

Allopathic treatment of obesity is carried out in phases, simultaneously or successively. The purpose is not only losing the weight but to treat the underlying ailment and preventing complications.

1. Treatment of Underlying Cause

i. *Evaluation of the Cause:* Differential diagnosis is evaluated for weight on various parameters. The purpose is to diagnose the root cause of weight gain that is, if it is primary obesity or something else. Commonly this is done by examination and investigation. Examination gives a primary idea about the possible underlying causes associated. Once it is confirmed a few laboratory or imaging investigations may be undertaken and diagnosis is confirmed.

ii. Once the diagnosis is confirmed, treatment of the cause is given according to medical guidelines. The medical treatment resolves disease and underlying cause.

iii. If there are multiple underlying causes, all the causes are taken care of in a planned manner. Some severe complications may be present or they may come up in the course of the treatment.

2. Treatment Specific to Weight Loss

i. Drugs for Appetite Suppression

There are three types of medicines:

- Noradrenergic agents
- Adrenergic agents
- Serotonin active agents

a. Noradrenergic Agents

Noradrenergic drugs such as derivatives of ephedrine depress the appetite center in hypothalamus and affect weight loss. They are mimetic of the sympathetic impulse in nature.

Drugs in this group include:

- Phenylpropanolamine
- Phentermine

Phenylpropanolamine:

- Dose: 75 mg taken once daily.
- Mimetic of the sympathetic impulse in nature.
- Directions: Under medical supervision.
- Adverse Effects: Nervousness, insomnia, dizziness, palpitations and headaches.

Phentermine (Ionamin):

- Similar to amphetamine and modulates noradrenergic neurotransmission to decrease appetite.
- Has little or no effect on dopaminergic neurotransmission.
- Dose 30.0 to 37.5 mg per day; phentermine is labeled for the management of exogenous obesity as short-term (that is, a few weeks) adjunct in a regimen of weight reduction based on caloric restriction.
- Adverse Effects: Headache, insomnia, nervousness and irritability, palpitations, tachycardia and elevation of blood pressure.

b. Adrenergic/Agents

Sibutramine:

- Inhibits monoamine uptake
- Suppressing appetite
- Thermogenesis from adipose tissue
- Dosage:
    - 10 mg once daily
    - Titrated to 15 mg, administered once daily if weight loss is adequate.

- Adverse Effects: Dry mouth, anorexia, constipation, insomnia, increase in blood pressure and heart rate.

Derivatives and free Leptin are also frequently used as appetite suppressant. The evidence of Leptin side effect is comparatively less as compared to other appetite control medications.

c. Serotonergic Agents:

Serotonergic drugs partially inhibit the reuptake of serotonin and release serotonins acting on the hypothalamus to decrease satiety.

Drugs in this group include

- Fenfluramine
- Dexfenfluramine
- Fluoxetine
    i. Serotonin reuptake inhibitor (SSRI)
    ii. Increase energy expenditure - raising basal body temperature

Fat Burners

Several fat burners are available with various compositions and contents. There are various claims and controversies in the same. Fat burners have major subgroups depending upon a few physiological functions:

i. Fat burners for men

ii. Fat burners for women

iii. Fat burners for diabetic patients

iv. Fat burners for athletes

Unfortunately, fat burners, despite having a lot of side effects on our body's physiology do not have much regulatory control. A few of such brand names are listed from A-Z in Appendix II.

Surgery

There are two different approaches. Surgery is usually indicated in severe or morbid cases where the weight is more than 45 kg above the normal upper limit. This may be indicated in cases having severe hypertension, sleep apnea, congestive cardiac failure, venous disease, etc.

i. Gastrointestinal tract intervention bypass:

   a. Jejunoileal bypass (least effective / almost abandoned).

   b. Vertical banded gastroplasty.

   c. Roux en Y gastric bypass.

Basically, all these three are appetite suppression treatments. This treatment will help reduce intake and reuptake.

Liposuction

Liposuction is surgery of fat remodeling. Also called lipectomy and lipoplasty. The surgery has received repute in recent days. This is done by removal of below skin fat by a stainless steel canula under a powerful vacuum.

Techniques of Liposuction:

- Dry liposuction
- Wet liposuction
- Super-wet liposuction
- Tumescent liposuction
- Laser assisted liposuction

Homeopathy

Homeopathy has a holistic approach to health. An obese constitution and the underlying cause or complication is treated by one single medicine that suits the entire person's constitution. Obesity is basically derived out of miasm and diathesis of some particular types.

Treatment of obesity from homeopathic point of view is one single medicine that covers the person's physical characteristics, mind set, symptoms and modalities. This medicine is selected on the similarity of all these essentials; called 'Simillimum'. Of late, there are many combinations marketed with homeopathic medicinces in them. These combinations include several homeopathically indicated drugs for obesity of which one may have a homeopathic effect on the problem while the others may produce their own side effects.

Common medicines used for treatment of obsesity in Homeopathy are Fucus vesiculosus, Calcarea carbonica, Thyreoidinum, Phytolacca, Capsicum, Graphites, Kalium bichromicum and Kalium carbonicum. Some medicines such as Ammonium carbonicum, Pulsatilla pratesus and Ferrum metallicum are also useful in this therapy. There are several other medicines very well suited to obese constitutions. There are about twenty different combinations available in the market for weight loss. The major physical action of most of these medicines is stimulation of hormones: Hypothalamic, pituitary and thyroid. Action of leptin on metabolism is per se not surely detectable due to lack of enough confirmation. Also, a fact that there cannot be generalisation of obesity medication, is worthy considering in this discussion.

Herbal Medicines / Ayurveda

Herbal medicines and the ayurvedic system of medicine are fantastic but unfortunately most misused for the control of obesity and weight loss. Generally, herbal medicines are known for helping weight gain. Yet, a few spices, some aperients and nutritives combine to produce excellent effects. The medicines in the list are guggulu (Commiphora mukul – gum resin), cinnamon, ginger, black / white pepper, lemon with water and honey, etc. Hirada alone or in combination with amla and behada (called triphala) is also one of the commonly known medicines for obesity and constipation.

Some commonly known herbal fat burners are green tea, lemon tea, mushrooms and lemon grass. All these in adequate quantity and in properly processed manner help reduce fats.

Ayurveda suggests replacement of sugar with honey – a fact tested by me too. Honey is sweeter than sugar and very low in sugar properties. Hence, in both these scenarios, honey helps in reduction of weight.

Counselling

Counselling is very important in all cases of obesity. The aim of counselling for obesity has various designs and reasons. Depending upon the stage in the course of treatment it has a lot to deliver.

1. **Counselling prior to treatment** The main aim of this counselling is to make the person understand the need to loose weight and complications of the treatment. Also, this counselling helps the person build self-confidence so that he or she can lose weight. The person should be convinced for the following things:

    i. There is no easier way of losing weight and losing weight is the necessity of the moment.

    ii. Determination is very important.

    iii. Set a realistic and achievable goal for weight loss and a time frame for the goal.

    iv. Treatment of any underlying psychological cause, if required, should be taken by the person.

2. **Counselling during the treatment tenure:**

    i. This counselling helps the person keep the confidence and efforts for weight loss up.

    ii. The aim for this counselling is also to console the patient's depression for not losing weight

Treatment of Obesity–Medicinal Therapy | 187

in the required proportion, not having significant changes in shape, anxiety arising from not having the liberty to eat and drink according to his own will or in converse, not having achieved the control on this, which is now becoming an impediment in the target to weight loss.

iii. In these counselling meetings, the patient should be helped to overcome his habits, intoxications, skipping of exercise habit, skipping of diet plan and habits. Lately, in case the patient is not able to lose weight, the counselling should also help the patient understand that his obesity is not treatable and he should not have any guilty feeling about the same.

3. Post-treatment / completion counselling:

i. There is only one, but complex aim of this counselling — inform the patient about his current status. Convince him about the status quo and instruct him about his behaviour in the future.

ii. In case the treatment has failed to achieve its targets, this counselling will help to restrict the depression of the patient.

Self-counselling is also possible as a substitute to all these counselling for various stages. This is very important to have a clear vision. Chalk out the self-counselling plan at the start of counselling itself, mainly considering the patient's habits and behavioural attitude. A very important matter of self-counselling is determination.

While concluding this chapter, we must take note of one thing that is, inevitably for all medicinal systems of – no medicine is free of side effects. Homeopathy and herbal medicines are many times considered to have no side effects. However, this is a misconception which usually leads to the abuse of medicines. Abuse, overuse and misuse of any medicine is always dangerous and sometimes even fatal. Hence, self-medication should be avoided strictly and all medication should be done strictly under medical observation only.

Review and Recap

Medical treatment has two aims in cases of obesity:

1. To treat the underlying disease.
2. To treat obesity and reduce weight.

Chapter 7

Complications of Obesity

The reason for all this detailed study and all this effort of interaction on obesity is in this chapter. Besides a chubby look affecting the cosmetic appearance, there are a lot of complications of obesity, some are even life threatening. Time and again, various small and big clinical researches have also revealed the relationship between obesity and various other illnesses, or at least, a very strong predisposition to such conditions. Let us understand these complications and ways to overcome the same.

Obesity and Cardiovascular Risks

Cardiac diseases have very high obesity related risk factors. Coronary heart disease, as per the American

Heart Association's study, has been found to have a direct co-relation with obesity, independent of other risk factors increased by obesity. These increased risk factors are high blood pressure, increased risk for diabetes, insulin resistance and increased blood cholesterol.

Women in their mid ages who are overweight, have an increased risk of cardiac disease by 50 per cent. This risk is augmented in males by about 72 per cent. This risk increases with the various factors discussed below:

Table 7.1

Parameter of Obesity	Intensity of Effect on Coronary (Ischemic) Heart Disease	Safe Range	High Risk Range, Very High Risk Range
BMI	Moderate	Men: 19 – 25 Women: 18 – 23	> 28 , > 35 > 26 , > 32
Waist size	High	Men: 94-101 cm Women: 80-87 cm	Non- Asian >= 102 cm Asian > = 90 cm Non –Asian > = 88 cm Asian > = 80 cm

(contd.)

(contd.)

Lying belly height	High	Men: Up to 23	23 – 25 , > 25
		Women: Up to 21	21 – 23, > 25
Waist to hip ratio	Moderate	Men: Up to 0.85	Men > 1.12
		Women: Up to 0.65	Women > 1.01
Fluctuating weight	Very high	No safe range	Fluctuation more than by 5 kg in 3 months

Other cardiac diseases are also prevalent in obese patients. Diseases such as left ventricular enlargement are commonly seen in obese patients. This may or may not be associated and linked with systemic hypertension. In most such cases, the ejection fraction is also lowered and the risk of congestive heart failure also increases. In the presence of obesity, if there is no systemic hypertension, left ventricular volume is often increased physiologically.

Risk of congestive heart failure is independently a complication of obesity as well. Increased stroke volume in the heart cycle, increased pumping effort and increased cardiac output is common in case of obesity. This leads either to increased systemic blood pressure or increased risk to heart failure. Conditions such as diastolic dysfunction of the left heart are also common in obesity, which many a times remains undiagnosed.

The risk of cardiac illness with the above three conditions turns fatal with or without diabetes in the form of cardiomyopathy, especially dilated.

Risk for other cardiovascular conditions also increases by up to 50 per cent in the presence of obesity. These diseases or conditions are systemic, pulmonary, postural and general hypertension, concentric left ventricular hypertrophy without dilatation, pulmonary embolism, hypoplastic coronary artery disease and arrhythmia. In a nutshell, all fatal diseases of the heart and circulation are predisposed with obesity and obesity increases its risk at least by 50 per cent.

Metabolic Complications of Obesity

Metabolic diseases and obesity have a very close relation. Diabetes and obesity is a known fatal combination, usually very common to occur. The constituents of a 'Metabolic syndrome' are increased lipids in blood (hyper cholesterolemia), insulin resistance or diabetes or both, increased triglycerides, increased plasma adiponectin (an enzyme acting on adipose tissue) and commonly adiposity of the abdomen. Central, especially abdominal fat increases the risk of metabolic syndrome several times.

Metabolic complications of diabetes are more common in the presence of obesity. These complications include ketosis, acidosis, insulin resistance, hyperglycemia and hypoglycemia in the morning. There is a several fold augmented risk of metabolic stress on liver in obesity, especially central abdominal obesity.

Blood lipid (Cholesterol) Abnormalities

Most commonly seen with obesity, being even 5 kg overweight can have such a complication. The lipid profile of an obese person is usually morbid. HDL (high density lipids) cholesterol is usally low in obesity, which increases all metabolic and cardiac risks further, where as triglycerides progressively increase to augment the risks.

Cancers/Tumours

The risks of certain cancers increase in obesity. These cancers are: Cancer of uterus, cervix, ovaries, breast, large intestines, rectum and prostate gland. This may be from various hormonal and metabolic reasons, but obese people are surveyed to have a higher risk for these cancers. Other tumours such as lipomas are also common in obesity.

The risk of cancers is separate in both sexes and various ages. In men, an increase in the BMI by 5, increases the risk of food pipe (oesophagus) cancer by more than 50 per cent. The risk of thyroid cancer is increased by almost one third times and cancer of kidneys by about one fourth times. In females, apart from the risk of increased breast cancer, there are increased risks by one or two third times towards gall bladder cancer, one third times to colon and rectum cancer and more than 50 per cent towards adenocarcinoma and almost 35 per cent towards cancer of the kidneys.

The risk for other cancers such as Non-Hodgkin's lymphoma, malignant melanoma (men) and pancreatic carcinoma (women) are also seen to be common. The overall likelihood of increased risk to cancer in the presence of obesity is 22–38 per cent.

Obesity and Liver Diseases

Besides the liver being overstressed, the risk of following hepatic and gall bladder conditions is also definitely increased by obesity.

1. Gall stones, especially of cholesterol type
2. Cholecystitis with or without stones.
3. Non-alcoholic fatty liver disease.

Risk for liver and gall bladder conditions increase by about 25 per cent overall and for the above three conditions, the risk augmentation is about double over, for the non-obese population. There are several evidences of liver cirrhosis increasing in obese women, especially in pork and beef eaters.

Gynecological Risks in Obesity

Gynecological problems related to obesity are more pertaining to the hormonal and structural impact. Fertility related conditions such as infertility, sterility are more common in obese women than in lean women. This risk is not studied per se, yet some informal papers report augmentation of 10 -15 per cent risk with overweight women.

Menstrual complaints such as irregular periods, suppressed menses, excessive bleeding, difficulty in menopause and painful menstruation have but unconfirmed risk augmentation. Considering the overall impact of obesity on menstruation, it pertains more to discomfort and the structural difficulty to manage. The number of women undergoing therapeutic curettage, Caesarian section and hysterectomy are more in the obese group than in the leaner group. Yet, this data needs confirmation by proper studies.

Other Risks

1. *Mental Depression:* Mental depression is common in obesity either from look, restricted physical activity or from any such social botheration or from any other unknown cause.

2. *Osteoarthritis:* Especially of the knees is more common in obese people, particularly women. This may be pertaining to the weight bearing proportion, but there is an overall risk augmentation by about 70 per cent.

3. *Skin problems:* Acne, intertrigo, delayed wound healing, varicosity, etc. are commonly seen more in case of obese people. There is a theory of accumulation of 'toxins' by naturopathy, which can possibly address and reason-out this complication better. This risk increase in obesity for skin problems is about 50 per cent.

4. *Sleep Apnea:* Peak-witchian syndrome, snoring and gasping breath in sleep.

Medication Related Risks

To be very frank, the treatment, rather the medical treatment of obesity has more risks of complication than obesity itself. There are several products, both edible and external that are available in the market at all points of time. Everyone makes a lot of promises and brings forth big dreams. But finally one needs to understand that, had all these things been so effective, obesity would not be the most incident non-communicable human disease.

The risks related to medication pertain to metabolism, injuries, accidents, cardiac arrest/arrhythmias, etc. Careful management of obesity with proper medical guidance is vitally important. The possibility of dietary imbalance, a non-carbohydrate diet, metabolic neurastnenia, etc. are seen to be very high in the condition of obesity.

Psychological Complications of Obesity and its Treatment

In most cases, the most ignored part in the treatment of obesity is counselling. In the absence of counselling, depression and panic are more common, which may later continue causing complications such as hysteria. All this is a matter of care and concern. There are people who take self-medication or self-treatment. They are known to have developed complications such as anorexia nervosa, etc. Anorexia nervosa is a condition where the person starves to reduce his/her weight and at the same time purging by misusing laxatives and emetics. In severe cases, they may have severe malnutrition and sometimes even dehydration. Anorexia nervosa also has some emergencies coming in like salt and water depletion, severe dehydrations and electrolyte imbalance.

Review and Recap

Complications of obesity are at various planes and the most common of them are psychological, cardiac and metabolic.

Chapter 8

50 Don'ts of Obesity – The Way to Avoid Obesity and its Related Complications

1. **Do not overeat**

   Availability of more than required food and the driven energy is responsible for adding fat bulk to the body. Whatever food is eaten in excess turns into fat. Ideally a person should eat only half of what is required to quench his appetite. The remaining half should be filled in with low energy fillers like roughage.

2. **Do not starve**

   Starvation is a known factor to stimulate fat accumulation. In fact, people who first starve and then suddenly start to eat grow fat faster than regular over-eater. If you are suggested to eat less, then fasting should be a programmed diet control. The diet must have all nutrients in it.

3. **Do not skip any nutrients in the food**

    This is a very important part for obesity. Any nutrient in excess should not be consumed but care should be taken that all the nutrients and enough roughage is being eaten in a day. Special attention is required on vitamins and minerals, the micronutrients, which are likely to be ignored when self diet control is done.

4. **Do not eat junk food**

    Junk food is the biggest cause from all angles for obesity. Junk food contains the least amounts of nutrients, has fat and carbohydrate content and is very low in roughage. This is a perfect combo for constipation, fat deposition and malnutrition.

5. **Do not consume excessive fats**

    Foods that contains cheese, oil, ghee, animal fats, cream, etc. have a lot of fat that accumulates in your body. If you are already obese, you need to refrain from eating all these. If you are not obese but tend to gain weight, watching your intake of these materials is a must.

6. Do not consume liquor

Liquor, especially, low to moderate concentrations alcoholic beverages are known to cause obesity. This is due to many things associated with them. Also, these beverages are usually served with snacks, which further increase our calorie intake.

7. Do not make a non-exercising life

Exercise is a must for a healthy being. A non-exercising life leads to obesity and many heart and lung diseases. If not possible for long, walk at least for fifteen minutes after both meals. If you are already obese, you need to increase your exercise to a level that some extra calories are also burnt every day.

8. Do not perform very fast exercise

Fast exercises help strengthen your heart and lungs, but it is hardly an aid to reduce weight. Calories are burnt in slow and initial exercises. The fat consuming exercises should cause a vibration of the obese parts and should also make one sweat off and on.

9. Do not leave scheduled exercises abruptly

A sudden stopping of exercises leads to deposition of fats in the areas which had highest exercise. If it is not possible to follow the whole schedule, at least stimulate the muscles of that area. Suddenly stopping exercise leads to extreme fat deposition in the areas which were being stretched in the exercise time.

10. Do not leave your belly loose after exertion and heavy meals

Often, some meals may be heavy. Also, after exercise, the belly muscles have a tendency to get remodeled. In all these cases, if the belly is left loose, it will take an obese shape. Hence, tie your tummy tightly after these two things. The whole tummy should be well tied, so that no part of it bulges.

11. Do not take aerated drinks

Aerated drinks contain lot of chemicals and sugar which hamper metabolism. Anything that is bubbling out is restricted according to ancient medicines. In case one needs to take these drinks, one must avoid black drinks that is, the cola flavours. Phosphoric acid in these black drinks is most harmful.

12. Do not consume canned foods and foods containing preservatives

Preservatives such as sodium meta bi-sulphate and vinegar have a metabolic impact. They interfere with the stimulation of adrenergic receptors. They also cause metabolic stress on the body.

13. Do not consume vinegar containing foods

Pure vinegar is known to reduce fat in large quantities. Glacial vinegar was being taken by Chinese people for reducing their fats; they consumed almost a small wine glass full of it. In spite of this, studies have shown that foods flavoured or seasoned with vinegar play a role in fat deposition.

14. Do not consume ajinomotto

Chinese or some continental and Thai foods having ajinomotto are known to cause quick and central obesity. This may or not have a direct relation with ajinomotto. Yet, it is always better to have healthier food.

15. Do not stress yourself

Physical and mental stress leads to increased steroidal secretion. Steroids are known to cause obesity. Mental stress also leads to some other conditions such as constipation and malnutrition, which, in turn, adds to obesity.

16. Do not consume steroidal medicines

Steroidal medicines are not uncommon in the Asian and Indian scenario, where some malpractices are also prevalent. One should be careful about consuming steroids. Chronic inflammatory conditions such as asthma, bronchitis, skin diseases, rheumatic arthritis involve steroidal therapy in their treatment. One must be skeptical about these treatments.

17. Do not misuse hormonal pills

Hormonal pills, especially estrogen and progesterone pills are used as oral contraceptives. Nowadays, there are some emergency contraceptives available in the market which contain hormones. There are also some pills for manipulating the menstrual cycle. They are also hormone based. These pills are known to cause fat deposition due to their hormonal action.

18. Do not smoke

Though smoking does not have a direct relation with obesity, it increases the risk of obesity related problems especially heart and vascular complaints. Smoking also leads to various issues of metabolism in diabetics. Therefore, smoking is always avoidable in all circumstances.

19. Do not eat non-vegetarian food

Food of animal origin is known to increase fats and causes deposition of fat in all risky areas.

20. Do not sleep immediately after eating

Sleeping immediately after eating is known to increase fat deposition. In a casual survey done on 200 obese people, 183 of 200 have or had the habit of sleeping immediately after eating.

21. Do not take a bath within one hour of eating

Flow of blood in the gastrointestinal tract is enriched during the digestive period. Vigorous activities such as bathing divert this flow, thereby slowing down absorption and thus leading to constipation, poor absorption and central obesity.

22. Do not discontinue steroids suddenly

Steroids should be tapered off, if at all, they are required to be taken in some conditions. This will help the body to gradually match the changes in the hormone levels of the body.

23. Do not consume medication without medical advice

Self-medication and non-medico prescribed medications are to be avoided. Various preparations in the market claim to reduce obesity. All these medications or weight loss preparations may tend to have a severe metabolic effect and may also cause secondary obesity.

24. Do not stop medication without proper monitoring and consultation

Withdrawal of medication against or in the absence of medical advice is more dangerous than starting such medication. When medication is withdrawn abruptly, its effect is more of a problem. The medication for lipid control, diabetes and thyroid treatment is strong at this point.

25. Do not hesitate to visit a psychiatrist or a psychologist

In case of psychiatric complaints or conditions that require psychological consultation; see a psychiatrist or psycho-therapist. Conditions like bulimia and obsessive compulsive disorder mandatorily seek these kind of advises.

26. Do not ignore signs of increasing weight

Do not ignore the signs of increasing weight such as a feeling of heaviness, difficulty in breathing from exertion, difficulty in rising from a seat, etc. These signs are elementary important features of primary fat depositions. When the signs are at this stage, contingency measures are still available.

27. Do not ignore symptoms such as swelling, appetite changes and cracks in heels

These symptoms may indicate underlying clinical conditions related to kidney or liver complaints. Proper investigation and treatment of these conditions must be done as early as possible. Proper treatment of these conditions in time will also help in quick recovery.

28. Do not have a fatty diet in post-surgical and post-parturition

Post-parturition and post-surgical period is a state of high energy liberation and at the same time very low physical activity. Apart from healing and restoration of physiological states, there are no primary energy utilising activities. Fat consumption during this period will lead to deposition of fat and constipation.

29. Do not consume a lot of sugar

Excess sugar and carbohydrates ultimately get converted into fats and lead to hypertrophy and hyperplasia of adipose cells. Increased adipose tissue increases fat in general. Sugar is the main content of sweet preparations, canned beverages, milk, tea, coffee, cappuccino, etc. Chocolates are also an important consideration. Honey should be given a preference over sugar.

30. Do not consume icy cold foods or beverages

Icy cold beverages, foods and even water are known to have a fat deposition effect. Even if there is no perfect mechanism known, this fact is accepted by many dieticians. Ice creams, jellies, canned juices or stored fresh fruit juices, cold water are the leading articles in this list.

31. Do not constipate

Avoid constipation. If you already suffer from the same, clearing bowels by taking a lot of roughage especially green leafy vegetables is essential. Drink more water and do adequate exercise. Constipation will lead to distension of abdomen and gradually central obesity.

32. Do not be pessimistic, depressed or anxious

Negative thoughts are known to cause and aggravate obesity. This also has a psychiatric correlation of hormones and the mental condition. Increased steroids due to a pessimistic attitude contributes to obesity or its reduction.

33. Do not eat stale food

Stale food without reprocessing is a heavier material. This will lead to fat deposition and a sluggish digestion rather than nutrition. It is said that stale food has more calories as all its micronutrients get destroyed and are converted into accumulating fat. Though this statement is not scientifically verified, may be true.

34. Do not eat farinaceous foods

All farinaceous foods have a high carbohydrate content. These foods take a lot of time to be digested and they also form a sticky mass in the abdomen. They cause constipation and flatulence. Like any other carbohydrate rich food, they also add to the conversion to fat.

35. Do not intermit the exercise

Intermitting exercise is counterproductive. If you have discontinued exercise, do not restart it unless you are determined to continue it religiously.

36. Do not depend on calorie count cynically

Calorie count actually creates panic rather than reducing weight. A better alternative is taking a balanced diet with programmed modifications. Any programmed modification will gradually but permanently reduce weight.

37. Do not make too austere a plan

Austere plans especially regarding food are usually very vulnerable and one soon gets bored and leaves them. Instead one should make a plan from which one does not get bored and is least likely of being left. Such a plan should also be well routed and flexibile.

38. Do not be irregular in medication

Medication in case of treatment of an underlying disease is an important part. Resistance to medication is common with obesity, especially insulin resistance. Avoiding this problem is partially possible with regularity of medication.

39. Do not forget updating the diet chart

If you are on a diet therapy, regularly updating your diet chart is vital. Following this practice religiously makes it possible to route, flex, modify and adjust diet characteristics.

40. Do not skip the regular check up

A regular check up of various constituents is very important in case of obesity. Cholesterol, blood sugar and any known other factor is vitally important. It is better to make a regular health record. Obesity is the seat for many diseases including heart complaints and diabetes. The risk of these diseases can be reduced by such regular monitoring.

41. Do not try to lose weight too quickly

Too quick a loss of weight may lead to problems and many a times some serious adverse conditions such as keto acidosis results. Weight loss should be a slow and steady programmed phenomenon.

42. Do not panic

Many people become panicked regarding their weight and increasing body size. Panic is the worst situation to be in. Stable treatment under medical watch is a viable alternative.

43. Do not get nervous

Nervousness increases conditions such as bulimia nervosa or at the same time may induce anorexia nervosa. Nervousness is an additional risk for depression which is an emotional cause of obesity.

There may be stress due to nervous behaviour. Hence, changing the pessimistic attitude and nervous temperament is the foremost step.

44. Do not hesitate to share your complaints and feelings

Many a times complaints and personal feelings regarding appetite, bowel movements, etc. are not shared with others due to modesty. This creates an obstacle in proper treatment. Hence one must share all the problems they face—symptoms, signs, feelings, everything.

45. Do not take excessively salty and full fat diet

This makes one vulnerable for hypertension, a commonly found condition with obesity. Salt restriction may not be needed unless there is an advanced pathology, but there should not be a well planned prevention strategy.

46. Do not over-medicate

Over-medication amd self-medication are counterproductive. A reasonably good number of advertisements and websites are now available which show the tendency of people to go for over-medication and self-medication for this reason. Obesity may or may not be a disease itself. But in both cases, it can lead to diseases, natural or induced.

47. Do not induce purging or vomiting

Induction of purging or vomiting is commonly seen in many patients. This may be due to some psychiatric condition such as bulimia nervosa or this may be out of hypochondriasis. These patients are observed to often suffer from water depletion and dehydration many times.

48. Do not ignore newly developed snoring habits

A newly developed snoring habit may indicate metabolic sleep apnea. A common example of this is Pick-witchian syndrome. If the snoring habit has developed recently, consult a physician and a sleep study specialist.

49. Do not take high calorie fruits

Ripe mangoes and bananas are fruits very rich in free fructose. Fructose will get converted to fat directly. Thus these fruits increase weight. While taking the fruits, one must be careful of their contents. These high calorie fruits should occupy less volume in the diet.

50. Do not experiment on yourself

As a lot of products, medicines, equipments, instruments are available in the market and getting advertised, it automatically makes one try one thing or another. This experimentation is harmful. No treatment for any disease is meant to be universal. The advertisements demonstrate their universal effect and superiority over the others. Yet, all these experiments are commercially inspired. Please take a proper consultation and go with classical treatment. Please remember, there is no option to diet control in the treatment of obesity.

Chapter 9

Appendix I – Conditions Including Obesity, Overweight and Weight Gain

Condition	Obesity type
Cortisone reductase deficiency	Abdominal obesity
Metabolic syndrome	Abdominal obesity, obesity
Borjeson syndrome	Adult obesity
McKusick kaufman syndrome – a type metaphyseal chondrodysplasia	Adult obesity
Prolidase deficiency	Childhood obesity
Lowe syndrome (oculocerebrorenal syndrome)	Chubby during younger years

(contd.)

(contd.)

Adrenal cortex neoplasms	Excessive body fat in torso
Adrenal gland hyperfunction	Excessive body fat in torso
Hyperadrenalism	Excessive body fat in torso
Cushing's syndrome	Obesity
Hyperpituitarism	Obesity
Achard-Thiers syndrome	Obesity
Albright like syndrome	Obesity
Albright's syndrome	Obesity
Ampola syndrome	Obesity
Aromatase deficiency	Obesity
Atkin-Flatiz syndrome	Obesity
Ayazi syndrome	Obesity
Bardet-Biedl's syndrome	Obesity
Bearn-Kunkel syndrome	Obesity
Biemond syndrome type II	Obesity
Bobble-head doll syndrome	Obesity
Carpenter's syndrome	Obesity
Chondrodysplasia, Grebe type	Obesity
Choroideremia	Obesity
Chromosome 11p, partial deletion	Obesity
Chromosome 12p, tetrasomy syndrome	Obesity
Chromosome 21q, deletion syndrome	Obesity

(contd.)

(contd.)

Chromosome 3, trisomy 3q13 2 q25	Obesity
Chromosome 4, trisomy 4p	Obesity
Chromosome 5, trisomy 5q	Obesity
Chromosome 5q, duplication syndrome	Obesity
Chromosome 9, partial trisomy 9p	Obesity
Clark-Baraitser syndrome	Obesity
Cohen Syndrome	Obesity
Del (1) (pter-p36)	Obesity
Del (2) (pter-p24) and dup (18) (q21-qter)	Obesity
Del (2) (q37)	Obesity
Del(1) (pter-p35)	Obesity
Deletion 6q16 q21	Obesity
Emerinopathy	Obesity
Empty sella syndrome – acquired	Obesity
Empty sella syndrome – primary	Obesity
Frolich's syndrome	Obesity
Fructose-1,6-bisphosphatase deficiency, hereditary	Obesity
Grahmann's syndrome	Obesity
Growth hormone receptor deficiency	Obesity
HAIR-AN syndrome	Obesity

(contd.)

(contd.)

Hydrocephalus obesity hypogonadism	Obesity
Hyperandrogenism	Obesity
Hyperostosis frontalis interna	Obesity
Hypertrichosis brachydactyly obesity and mental retardation	Obesity
Hypogonadism – mitral valve prolapse – mental retardation	Obesity
Hypogonadotropic hypogonadism -- syndactyly	Obesity
Laron pituitary dwarfism	Obesity
Leschke-Ullmann syndrome	Obesity
Mauriac syndrome	Obesity
Metaphyseal dysostosis – mental retardation – conductive deafness	Obesity
MOMO syndrome	Obesity
Nguyen syndrome	Obesity
Leptin deficiency	Obesity
Polycystic ovarian disease, familial	Obesity
Prader-Willi syndrome	Obesity
Retinohepatoendocrinologic syndrome	Obesity
Schinzel syndrome	Obesity
Schroeder syndrome 1	Obesity

(contd.)

(contd.)

Sengers-Hamel-Otten syndrome	Obesity
Sohval-Soffer syndrome	Obesity
Subaortic stenosis – short stature syndrome	Obesity
Summitt syndrome	Obesity
Urban Rogers Meyer syndrome	Obesity
Vasquez Hurst Sotos syndrome	Obesity
WAGR syndrome	Obesity
Wilms tumour	Obesity
Wilson-Turner X-linked mental retardation	Obesity
X-linked mental retardation craniofacial abnormal microcepahly club	Obesity
Young Hughes syndrome	Obesity
Adrenal cancer	Obesity, excessive body fat in torso
Weight cycling	Obesity, Overweight
Eating disorders	Obesity, Weight gain
Polycystic ovarian disease	Obesity, weight gain
Chromosome 1, uniparental disomy 1q12 q21	Overweight
Chromosome 1p deletion syndrome	Overweight
Lipoprotein disorder	Overweight

(contd.)

(contd.)

Hypothalamic dysfunction	Overweight, increased weight
Klinefelter syndrome	Rounded body type, overweight

Appendix II – Fat Burners

	Extreme Acai Berry	**Nustevia**
AbGone	Fastin	Nutriveda
Acai Berry Detox	Fat Loss 4 Idiots	NV Review
Acai Berry Power 500	Fat Stripper	Oral HCG Diet Solution
Acai Berry Select	Force Factor	PGX Daily
Acai Body Flush	Formula Pi2	Pheninol
Acai Elite	Lemon Maple Syrup Cleanse	Phenocal
Acai Fuel Extreme	Leptorexin	Phenocerin
Acai Noni Burner	Leptovox	Phenolox
Acai Slim (AcaiSlim)	Levorex	Phenphedrine
AcaiPure	Life Cleanse	Phenterdrene p 57
Accomplix	Life Extension Integra-Lean Irvingia	Phentermine
Accomplix Burn	Lipaphen RX	Phenterpril
Accomplix Carb	Lipo-6	Phenterthin

(contd.)

(contd.)

Accomplix H2O	Lipo-6 Black	Phentirmene
Adapexin	Lipo-6 Hers	Phentrazine Slimcaps
Adipex	Lipo-6x	Phosphacore
Adipozil	Lipofuze	Pomclear
Adipozin	Lipolyze	Power Flush 500
Adipril	Liporexall	Primal Force Primal Lean
Advanced Acai	Liposlim	Proactol
All Natural Body Flush	Lipovox	Probiotic Complete
Alli	Lipovox Hardcore Detox	QuickTrim Fast-Shake
Allure Patch	FucoSlim	Rapidcuts Hardcore
Amfedrine	Fucoxanthin Formula 1332	Redline Energy Drink
Amphedrine	Fucozan	Reduslim
Anoretix	Fullbar	Ronaxil
Apatrim	Fullbites (by Fullbar)	RX6 45 Capsules by BPI
Atro Phex	Garden Greens Acai Blast	SlendeSlim
Avesil	Garden of Life Fucothin	Slendrex
Awe Slim	Glucotrin	Slim 365
Banitrim	GNC X-12	Slim Chews

(contd.)

(contd.)

BetaStax	Green Tea Extreme	Slim Easy
Blue Print Cleanse	Green Tea Fat Burner Plus	Slim4Life
Body Trim	Hoodia Gordonii Plus	Slimburst
BPI Sports 1MR	Hoodia Stack	SlimQuick
Bromalite	IdealCleanse Diet	SlimQuick Cleanse
Burn the Fat Feed the Muscle	IntraCleanse	SlimShots
CalmSlim	Irvingia Gabonensis	SlimSplash
Caltrap	Irvingia Plus	Slimunique
Celerite	Jillian Michaels EXTREME Maximum Strength Calorie Control	SomnaSlim
Century Systems The Cleaner	Jillian Michaels EXTREME Maximum Strength Fat Burner	South Beach Acai
Clinicallix	Jillian Michaels QUICKSTART Rapid Weight Loss Program	Stemulite

(contd.)

(contd.)

CocoTrim	Jillian Michaels Triple Process Detox and Cleanse Plus Probiotic Replenishment	Strip That Fat
Coloflush	Kintopill	The Ice Cube Diet
Cologenix	Lean System 7 Clinical Strength	Thermo Lean
Colon Flow	Leangenix	Think and Lose
Colon xR	Max WLX	TopRatedFatBurners.com
Colon700	Medifast	TrimSlim
Colotrim	Mega T Green Tea	TrimSpa
Control ACS	Mega T Green Tea Chewing Gum	Ultra Lean Green Tea
CST Boost	Metabolife Aquaslim	Ultra Strength Taraxatone Extreme
Curvatrim	Metabolife Break Through	USPLabs Recreate
Curvelle	Metabolife Caffeine Free	Venom Hyperdrive
Cytolean V2	Metabolife Extreme Energy	VitalAcai
DecaSlim	Metabolife Green Tea	VPX Meltdown

(contd.)

(contd.)

DecaTrim	Metabolife Ultra	Waterex
Deep Diet Pill	Methyl Ripped	WeightLossDiet.net
Detoxykall	MiracleBurn	Wu Yi Tea
Dexatrim	MiracleBurn Cream	Wu-Yi Easy Weight Loss Tea
dietpilldiscounts.com	Napsil	Xellex
Dual Action Diet Cleanse	Natrol Carb Intercept	Xenadrine RFA-X
Dyma-Burn Xtreme	Natural Acai	Zantrex
Elite Hoodia	Natural Made Acai	Zotrim
Ephedra Hoodia Fusion	Nitetrim	
Ephedrasil Hardcore	Noxycut	
Estrin-D	Nuphedragen	

Appendix III – Calorie Content of Common Food Material

Cereals	Energy per 100 grams	Cereals	Energy per 100 grams
Bagel	310	Pasta (normal, boiled)	110
Biscuits	480	Pasta (whole wheat, boiled)	105
Jaffa cake	370	Porridge-oats (with water)	55
Bread–white	240	Potatoes (boiled)	70
Bread–whole wheat (thick)	220	Potatoes (roast)	140
Chapattis	300	Rice (white)	140
Cornflakes	370	Rice (brown)	135
Cream crackers	440	Rice cakes	373

(contd.)

(contd.)

Crumpets	198	Ryvita multi grain	331
Flapjacks–basic fruit mix	500	Ryvita + seed and oats	362
Macaroni (boiled)	95	Spaghetti (boiled)	101
Muesli	390	Sorghum (jawar) bread	260
Naan–bread (normal)	320	Sorghum (bajra) bread	330
Noodles (boiled)	70		
Fruits and Vegetables	**Energy per 100 grams**	**Fruits and Vegetables**	**Energy per 100 grams**
Apple	44	Mushrooms–raw (one average)	15
Banana	65	Mushrooms (boiled)	12
Beans–baked beans	80	Mushrooms (fried)	145
Beans–dried (boiled)	130	Olives	80
Blackberries	25	Onion (boiled)	38
Blackcurrant	30	Onion–red (one)	53

(contd.)

(contd.)

Broccoli	32	Onions–spring	25
Cabbage (boiled)	20	Onion (fried)	155
Carrot (boiled)	25	Orange	30
Cauliflower (boiled)	30	Peas	148
Celery (boiled)	10	Peas–dried and boiled	120
Cherry	50	Peach	30
Courgette	20	Pear	38
Cucumber	10	Pepper, yellow	16
Dates	235	Pineapple	40
Grapes	62	Plum	39
Grapefruit	32	Spinach	8
Kiwi	50	Strawberries (one average)	30
Leek (boiled)	20	Sweetcorn	130
Lentils (boiled)	100	Tomato	20
Lettuce	15	Watercress	20
Melon	28		

(contd.)

(contd.)

Poppers	Energy per 100 grams	Poppers	Energy per 100 grams
Animal fat - including ghee and butter	900	Mars bar	480
Bombay mix	500	Mints	100
Butter	750	Oils–corn, sunflower, olive	900
Chocolate	500	Popcorn– average	460
Cod liver oil	900	Sugar–white, table sugar	400
Corn snack	500	Sweets (boiled candies)	300
Crisps (chips US) average	500	Syrup	300
Honey	280	Toffee	400
Jam	250	Sweetcorn on the cob	70
Lard	890	Tomato– cherry	17
Low fat spread	400	Tomato puree	70
Margarine	750		

(contd.)

(contd.)

Milk Products	Energy per 100 grams	Milk Products	Energy per 100 grams
Cheese–average	440	Eggs (fried)	180
Cheddar types–average, reduced fat	260	Fromage frais	125
Cheese spreads–average	270	Ice cream	180
Cottage cheese–low fat	80	Milk–whole	70
Cottage cheese	98	Milk–semi-skimmed	50
Cream cheese	428	Milk–skimmed	38
Cream–fresh half	160	Milk–soya	36
Cream–fresh single	200	Mousse flavored	140
Cream–fresh double	430	Omelette with cheese	266
Cream–fresh clotted	600	Trifle with cream	190
Custard	100	Yogurt–natural	60
Eggs (one, average size)	150	Yogurt–reduced fat	45